AF411478

Close to the Edge:
Brånemark and the Development of Osseointegration

Close to the Edge

Brånemark and the Development of Osseointegration

Elaine McClarence
London, England

Quintessence Publishing Co. Ltd.
London, Berlin, Chicago, Copenhagen, Paris, Milan, Barcelona, Istanbul,
São Paulo, Tokyo, New Delhi, Moscow, Prague, Warsaw

British Library Cataloguing in Publication Data

McClarence, Elaine
  Close to the edge: Brånemark and the development of osseointegration
  1. Brånemark, Per-Ingvar 2. Osseointegration
  I. Title
  617.4'710592

  ISBN 185097067X

Copyright © 2003 by Quintessence Publishing Co. Ltd., London

Quintessence Publishing Co. Ltd.
Grafton Road, New Malden
Surrey, KT3 3AB, United Kingdom
www.quintpub.co.uk

All rights reserved. This book or any part thereof may not be reproduced, stored in a retrieval system, or transmitted in any form or by any means, electronic, mechanical, photocopying, or otherwise, without the written permission of the publisher.

ISBN 1-85097-067-X

Printed in Germany

Contents

Preface

I first met Per-Ingvar Brånemark on April 24, 1986. At the time, I was a journalist at the *Financial Times* in London, writing about developments in science and technology. Meeting Brånemark was an interesting experience. He was obviously suspicious of journalists, even those from reputable journals, and he did not enjoy answering inane questions from people who would probably not grasp the true significance of his work.

My audience with Brånemark was relatively short, and I recorded in my diary that he was "brilliant but evasive." He answered my questions patiently and then swept out of the room, leaving me to gather my notes and depart for London.

My article appeared in the Technology section of the *Financial Times* but was cut in half because my editor felt the descriptions of amputees would be too upsetting for our financial readers. I was incensed by this, and so I wrote a short but business-oriented article for another section of the paper that was not so drastically edited.

Four years later I received a call from Rune Davidsson, who worked at Brånemark's Institute for Applied Technology and was an intermediary between Brånemark and Nobelpharma (now Nobel Biocare), the business set up to make the titanium components and related equipment. Apparently Brånemark had liked my work – and could tolerate my presence – and a 25-year celebration of osseointegration was approaching and required some journalistic input.

Since that time, I have continued to work intermittently with Professor Brånemark on various projects. They always require that I stretch my intellect to its full capacity and delve into topics outside my normal sphere of writing. On one occasion, I shared with Dick Skalak, a long-time friend and colleague of Brånemark's, that medical writing was so far outside my experience that I felt I should leave it to others more qualified to do it. Dick smiled and replied that since Per-Ingvar respected my work and trusted me, there was little chance of my escaping this duty. The best thing was to buy a good medical book, continue to learn about osseointegration, and accept my fate with humor and good grace. This I have done. It has been a rewarding and enriching experience.

This book is intended to fulfill two conflicting goals. I wanted to provide a short, updated history of the development of osseointegration while, at the same time, providing some scientific and clinical background. The overall aim of this work is to serve as a general introduction for those embarking on the study of osseointegration and for those curious to know something about this fascinating technique.

There are many, many people I would like to thank, and the list would almost make a book of its own. I would like to thank the following people personally for their support, their willingness to give of their time, and their proofreading skills.

Much gratitude goes to Per-Ingvar Brånemark and his staff at the Institute: Barbro Svenson, Marianne Szabó, Rigmor Carlsson, Ylwa Winsnes Johansson, Elisabeth Gröndahl, and Rikard Brånemark. Thanks also to Christina Brånemark for her sage comments on the final manuscript.

The late Richard Skalak was a great support. I miss his humor, good advice, and insight into the tale of osseointegration.

Björn Rydevik and Ulf Nannmark have been generous with both their time and knowledge. Thanks also to Shu Chien, who has revealed much about the workings of cells in relation to osseointegration. I have learned much and appreciate their continued collaboration.

Finally, there are the many patients, clinicians, anaplastologists, doctors, and dentists with whom I have come into contact over the years. They are an inspiration.

Introduction

In May 1993, Per-Ingvar Brånemark and the late Richard Skalak wrote a short article about the state of osseointegration as they saw it at the time. For various reasons, this philosophical summary of the world of osseointegration was never published. But the passage of time has not dulled its relevance. It seems appropriate that those thoughts formulated almost a decade ago should find a home in this publication.

Osseointegration has been, and still is, a phenomenon subject to much debate, as well as research. Behind the nuances of semantics and the rigor of scientific scrutiny, the development of the concepts and practice of osseointegration has created a quiet revolution in dentistry and other restorative and orthopedic fields, with very favorable practical results. The perceived nature of the effects and challenges of this revolution varies with the role of the observer and the nature of his or her involvement, whether as patient, oral surgeon, prosthodontist, orthodontist, audiologist, orthopedist, plastic surgeon, scientist, engineer, scholar, or businessperson.

For the completely edentulous patient receiving a complete fixed prosthesis supported by osseointegrated implants, it has brought a level of function, security, permanence, and esthetic and psychological satisfaction that was previously impossible. The patient's satisfaction and function is the prime achievement of osseointegration. Furthermore, its applications to single-tooth and multiple-tooth situations, as well as its use in craniofacial, plastic surgery, and orthopedic situations, are still being explored and successfully expanded.

From the standpoint of medical practitioners as surgeons, prosthodontists, or general practitioners, the development of osseointegration has meant availability of a new treatment modality that is a challenge to understand and use and to consider using or adapting among many treatment modalities. It has not been a method that simply extends previous techniques. Osseointegration has required special training and new ways of thinking and practice. It has, thus, allowed a very sound and reliable new treatment to be carefully considered for each new patient.

For research scientists, biologists, and bioengineers, osseointegration has raised a series of interesting, often perplexing, and wide-ranging questions that have been rewarding to pursue insofar as answers have been developed. Many are still unanswered. The research questions start at a material level: What are the surface properties that enhance or inhibit osseointegration? Further, what form should an implant and prosthesis take? On the biological side, there are questions of a more difficult nature: What cells and matrix components are responsible for the success or failure of a fixture to integrate in bone? What factors affect integration? What are the controls and limits to the rate and strength of osseointegration? What immunological and soft tissue responses are needed or should be avoided? The total complexity of these fundamental biological questions is just now being unraveled through rigorous studies. The understanding and control of long-term changes due to bone resorption and/or growth and densification are not understood in detail and obviously involve complex cellular mechanisms of sensing and response. Molecular genetics and genetic engineering may even play a role.

From the standpoint of a manufacturer, the development of osseointegration presents challenges of optimization and precision control in production of a new line of products. For a complete and successful product line, new tools and equipment must be provided as well. Further, the production methods, material selection, and engineering designs being used today will not necessarily be optimal or practical in the future, so there is room for creative industrial innovation. In addition, training courses are necessary if the new products are to be successfully used. These requirements and their satisfaction have led to an entirely new industry, complete with regular and systematic training programs and university curricula to lead and train students in clinical procedures, patient selection, maintenance, handling of complications, and health care.

Finally, from the viewpoint of the science historian, socially minded commentator, or government administrator, osseointegration is a clear, classic example of advanced technology applied for the benefit of people's health instead of their destruction. It may be useful to consider the socioscientific structures and research-funding mechanisms that will best allow for similar new developments to arise and prosper in the future. From a historical viewpoint, the discovery and practical application of osseointegration has been an explosive event, a blink of the eye in an evolutionary timescale. But for those involved on a daily basis, it may seem, at times, to be a slow, difficult, and thorny road in practice. Perhaps there is no other way.

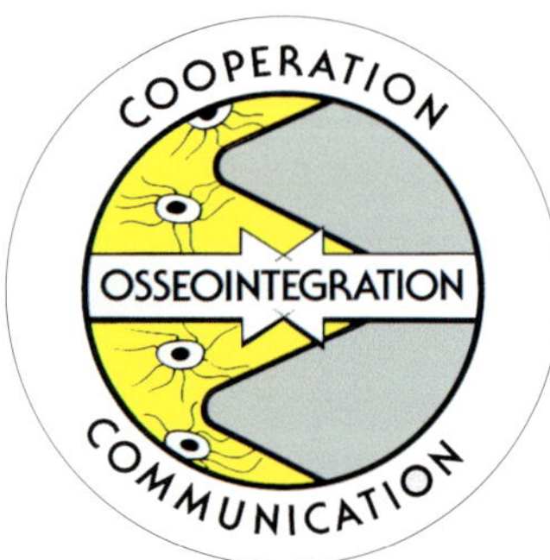

Fig 1   It was recognized early on that the success and growth of osseointegration was dependent on collaboration, cooperation, and communication between all the players in health care – researchers, clinicians, health care providers, and industry. This illustration embodies these ideals and communicates Brånemark's vision.

Historical Developments

Part I

1 Foundations

The work of Per-Ingvar Brånemark and his colleagues now has a history going back more than 40 years, so it is often difficult to comprehend how revolutionary this work was during the 1950s and 1960s.

Brånemark never set out to develop a method of bonding titanium components to bone. He was a researcher interested in the development of *in vivo* techniques to study the nature and behavior of blood. His early work, including his doctoral thesis, was carried out at Sweden's Lund University. It provided insights into blood circulation in bone and marrow.

Bone Biology

At the time Brånemark was involved in this research activity, no one knew much about the generation of new blood cells. Today, it is an established fact that red blood cell formation, hemopoiesis, is a vital process that takes place in red bone marrow. Such marrow is found in the spongy type of bone in the ends of some long bones. Spongy bones contain many spaces that may be filled with marrow.

Bones are complex structures. They are more than simply the scaffolding that supports and protects the organs and other body components. Within their seemingly solid construction is an intricate network of different types of bone material. The outer layer of bone is hard and dense and made up of a matrix organized into many structural components called Haversian systems. These systems are reminiscent of the layers of an onion and are created by layers of calcified matrix called lamellae. At the core of this tube-like structure is the Haversian canal, which contains a blood vessel (Fig 1-1). Spongy

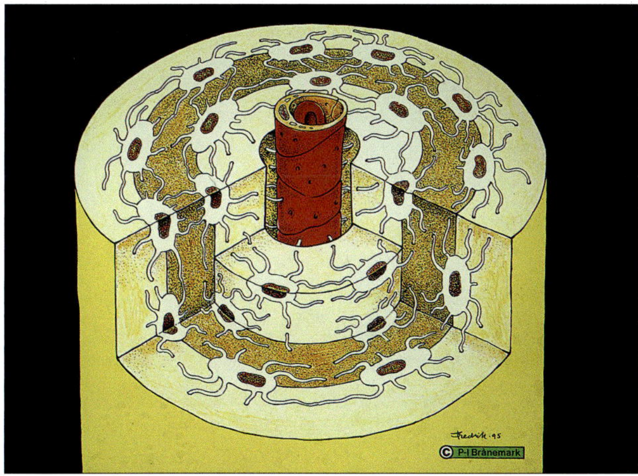

Fig 1-1 Schematic illustration of the anatomy of the Haversian system. Osteocytes are organized in layers surrounding the central vascular canal.

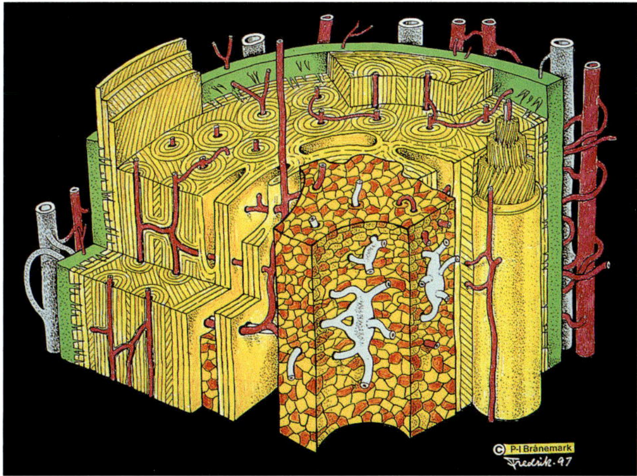

Fig 1-2 Bone is a complex, highly organized tissue, constantly changing in response to mechanical signals. It has a system of canals consisting of cell, cell processes, blood vessels, lymphatic vessels, and nerves permeating the bone matrix.

bone, by contrast, contains needle-like threads of bone that surround a network of spaces called trabeculae. The bone matrix also harbors a number of special cells with important functions. Osteocytes, living bone cells, lie trapped in spaces called lacunae found in the hard layers of the lamellae. Tiny passages or canals called canaliculi link osteocytes with each other and with the central canal in each Haversian system. The blood vessel at the center of each Haversian system delivers nutrients via the canaliculi to the osteocytes (Fig 1-2). In addition to the bone-forming osteocytes, specialized cells called osteoclasts are present in bone. These cells play a key function in bone repair and regeneration by removing damaged or unwanted bone. It is the combined efforts of bone-producing osteoblasts and bone-absorbing osteoclasts that fashion the skeleton into its final shape. It is not just in the early years of life that our bone structure needs to accommodate growth and change. Throughout our adult life, bone is reacting to changing conditions. It is one of the most dynamic materials in our body, not unlike the "shifting sands of time."

Early Experiments

Brånemark wanted to study the potential of bone to heal after injury and the way bone, marrow, and blood could interact. In particular, he was trying to establish a connection between healing and marrow mechanisms in bone. To this end, Brånemark devised a series of experiments that involved studying the marrow as it carried out its work during healing. To do this, he employed an inspection chamber that could be surgically inserted into living bone, in this case a rabbit fibula. These chambers could be connected to a specially adapted microscope to record and track the changes taking place in the bone. The development of the inspection chamber was in itself quite a challenge.

As he worked to identify the best experimental approach for his studies, Brånemark met with other researchers in the United Kingdom and the United States. While he was on a 2-week trip to the United Kingdom in the 1950s, he came in contact with some researchers at Cambridge University who had developed a special chamber to look at blood flow in rabbits. These chambers were inserted in the soft tissue of the ears. Brånemark was certain such chambers could be adapted so they could be used to study blood flow in bone, rather than soft tissue.

This is where the first small step toward osseointegration occurred. As a result of a shortage of engineering materials, Brånemark could not make the chambers from the metal tantalum as the Cambridge researchers had. He opted for titanium instead. The post-war era in Europe was a period in which exotic scientific materials were in short supply and consequently expensive and difficult to obtain. The global economy that existed in part prior to the Second World War had been completely destroyed, making acquisition of any special materials a mammoth task. Titanium ore is found in a number of countries including Canada, Russia, the United States, Malaysia, and Australia. In the early 1950s, titanium was little understood, and its uses were mainly unknown outside military and aerospace applications.

An English clergyman and amateur mineralogist, William Gregor, first noted the existence of titanium in 1791. It took more than 100 years to isolate the element itself, and commercial production of the pure metal required the development of a new melting technique. One of the main motivations to produce titanium is its strength combined with its light weight. Although it is a highly reactive element in its molten form, titanium as a solid is highly resistant to chemical attack. It is more resistant to corrosive substances than stainless steel, for example.

In 1948, a mere 3 tons of the metal were produced, but by the late 1980s, the quantity was in excess of 300,000 tons. The application of titanium is split almost evenly between the pure metal and a variety of alloys. Alloys are used in aircraft components, military equipment, and a range of industrial components such as steam turbine blades, crankshafts, and camshafts. It is the corrosion resistance of titanium – from chemicals and biological attack – that has made it attractive for use in steam turbine tubing, chemical production plants, and in biomedical applications. These attributes of pure titanium, along with other properties, have combined to make it highly suitable for osseointegrated components.

As Brånemark points out, however, titanium is not unique in its ability to exist without causing reaction within the human frame, and time and research may reveal other equally suitable materials. The pace of development of biocompatible materials is rapid, and there are a wide variety of materials from metal compounds to plastics to ceramics that can be used in clinical work today. Many scientists are looking at the interaction between biological tissues as artificial materials are introduced. A number of techniques are available that allow the observation, either directly or indirectly, of surface interactions at the molecular level. It is hoped that this may lead to a greater understanding of the nature of biocompatibility and the behavior of blood and tissue during the crucial moments when they come into contact with biomaterials.

In the late 1950s, however, little information was available outside the military on the workings of titanium. Special care was required. Titanium, though strong, is a relatively soft metal, which makes it difficult to machine. If extreme care is not taken, the metal can cause the cutting tool to heat up too rapidly and bits of titanium can stick to, or become welded to, the cutting head, which causes damage. If too many small particles build up at the workpiece, the metal can burst into flames. To successfully make precision components, machining has to be performed with high-quality, heat-resistant cutting tools operating at relatively low speeds to limit the amount of heat created during the process.

Having obtained titanium, Brånemark used the metal for the development of a titanium device that could be used for *in vivo* studies. The titanium chambers were used to a positive effect. The chamber was inserted into a rabbit fibula, as Brånemark believed this was the best site to watch the interaction between blood and marrow. Brånemark used a very delicate surgical procedure that caused minimal tissue injury to ensure he would be able to observe the events taking place. Any major damage to the tissue would obscure the repair mechanism taking place in the bone and marrow. Eventually, he saw blood cells being formed in the marrow. As it turned out, the osseointegration technique that was to develop from this work would rely on an equally sensitive surgical approach. The important lesson was that bone has only a limited capacity for repair and should be treated with the same respect that the more obviously delicate parts of the body, such as the eye and brain, receive.

Along with the excitement of this discovery, Brånemark also had a moment of panic while reading a scientific paper by another researcher. In it, the author stated that the conditions in the rabbit fibula were atypical, so any research involving that part of the animal's anatomy could not be applied to other parts of the skeleton. It spoiled the rest of Brånemark's evening. He spent a sleepless night worrying about the validity of 3 years' research. On returning to the laboratory the next day, he rechecked his data and reassured himself that all was well.

The experiments took several months to complete. Once they were over, Brånemark tried to retrieve the titanium chambers for reuse. These were expensive items and not easy to replace in the post-war university environment. Imagine his irritation when he found it was impossible to extract the device. As the chamber had been in situ for a considerable time, bone had grown into all the crevices and threads. The titanium chamber appeared to have become an integral part of the bone structure.

Brånemark, focused as he was on the blood and marrow studies, did not at this point make the next leap of discovery required for the story of osseointegration. On the contrary, he registered annoyance that a valuable component had been lost.

Professorship on Offer

In 1960, Per-Ingvar Brånemark became an associate professor at the age of 31 (Fig 1-3). He moved from Lund to Gothenburg to become professor of anatomy at that city's university. Originally, Gothenburg University had offered him a position in experimental surgery, but a second offer in the department of anatomy better suited him, as it offered the opportunity to continue his research. At Gothenburg, the nature of this research was to change somewhat. In many ways, it was a logical progression from the bone and marrow studies that had been carried out at Lund. Now Brånemark took an interest in blood circulation. The 1960s was a time of

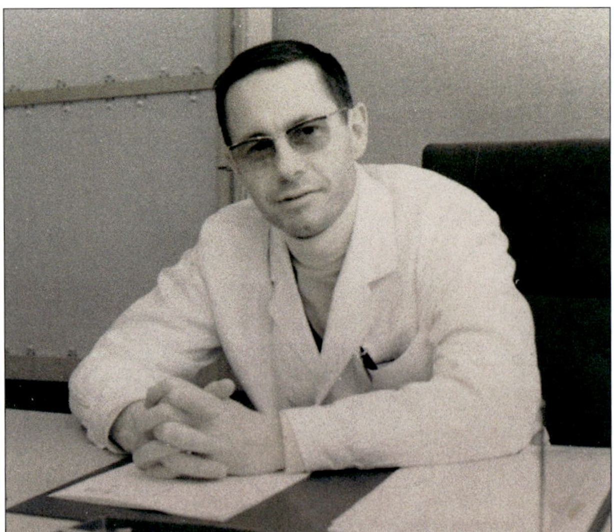

Fig 1-3 Brånemark as a young associate professor.

rapid development in imaging technology, including the development of more sophisticated light microscopes. Brånemark jokes that he had only been at Gothenburg University a week when he was asked if he had any ideas on how to spend some excess capital quickly before the money was lost. This was an easy task as Brånemark had some ambitious research plans. Brånemark's department managed to square the university's budget by acquiring some of the latest microscope technology, providing the essential resources needed for Brånemark's extensive research program.

In a relatively short time, Brånemark had initiated a huge body of research that drew in some of the best minds of their generation in Sweden. The newly formed Microcirculation Laboratory, based on the established reputation Brånemark brought from Lund, was a honey pot for students wishing to pursue careers in clinical research. Indeed, while Brånemark remained head of this laboratory, many researchers gained their doctorates and went on to become eminent professors in their own fields of expertise. More than 20 students produced their doctoral theses from their work at the laboratory while Brånemark was there.

University Experiments

One of the reasons this laboratory was so productive was that the research was broad and involved people from a number of disciplines. Later, this multidisciplinary collaboration would be of crucial importance in developing all aspects of the osseointegration work, even commercial introduction of components and instruments in the 1980s, as well as the basic clinical procedures.

Blood circulation studies, by this time, had revealed much about the nature and purpose of blood in human and animal anatomy. There were some gaps, however. In particular, Brånemark and his enthusiastic team of students intended to focus on the anatomy and function of blood corpuscles.

One of the main achievements of this work was to present films of blood flow moving through the microcirculation. Brånemark managed to produce clear-moving images recorded through the microscope that revealed the dynamic nature of blood and its interaction with surrounding vessels, as well as its constituent parts. These studies came to the attention of a young American researcher, Richard Skalak, when Brånemark gave a lecture on blood flow during a visit to Philadelphia. Skalak, an engineer, chose to spend a sabbatical year in Gothenburg, and this was the start of a long professional relationship between the two men, which continued until Skalak's death in 1997.

Brånemark's ability to use available technology to the best effect is due, in no small way, to the fact that he had always had a deep interest in engineering. At one point, he had considered an engineering, rather than a medical, career. This has always given him an interest in and respect for those working in fine mechanics and the development of technology. Living in both worlds also helped him realize that the future of osseointegration, once all the threads of the work were identified, lay in a multidisciplinary approach and would need to involve a number of people with different experiences and skills.

Another step in this direction came through the set of experiments devised for studying the blood flow. These involved using an adaptation of the titanium inspection chambers used in the previous bone and marrow research. In this case, however, the chambers were to be inserted in human subjects. Altogether, 17 volunteers, 14 male and 3 female (most of them Brånemark's students), agreed to have small chambers inserted in the underside of their upper arms (Fig 1-4). These chambers remained in situ for between 3 and 7 months, except in the case of one student who forgot about the chamber and went into a sauna, which caused tissue damage through burns since titanium is a good conductor of heat. The chamber had to be removed, though the student did not suffer any long-term effects, apart from embarrassment. This experiment aimed to provide a window to an isolated part of the human circulation. The basic principle of this experiment was to use a thin layer of vascularized tissue with parallel surfaces grown in a twin pedicle skin tube on the inside of the upper arm. This tissue was then enclosed between glass elements and secured by the titanium chamber. This window into human anatomy could then be connected to a light microscope that allowed detailed analysis of various morphologic and dynamic parameters related to the anatomy and rheology of blood in the nutritive, microvascular portion of the circulation system (Fig 1-5). To monitor the blood cell behavior, the volunteer would lie on his or her back on a table close to the microscope, but not connected to it. The left arm, which contained the implant, was supported on a stand mounted on a cross stage that enabled careful adjustment of the upper arm to avoid inappropriate stretching of the skin tube. The chamber was immobilized in a special holder, and the arrangement allowed illumination from below. As

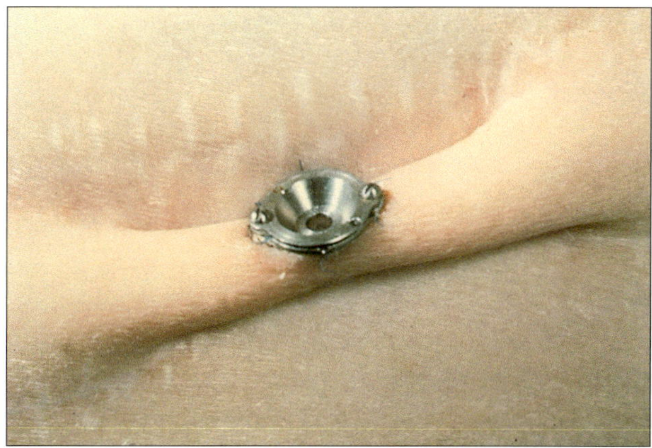

Fig 1-4 A small titanium inspection chamber was inserted in the upper arm of volunteers for the blood cell studies.

uncomfortable as this was for the volunteers, some had to endure further discomfort as the studies progressed.

Having established the basic behavior and anatomy of blood cells in their natural habitat, the next aim was to look at what happened when outside influences impinged on this environment. In practical terms, this meant an individual eating, drinking, or smoking while the observers charted what changes occurred in the microcirculation. One student participant, Göran Lundborg, now a professor in hand surgery at Lund University, ate 500 g of butter. Despite this experience, Lundborg remains a close scientific collaborator with Brånemark. Under the

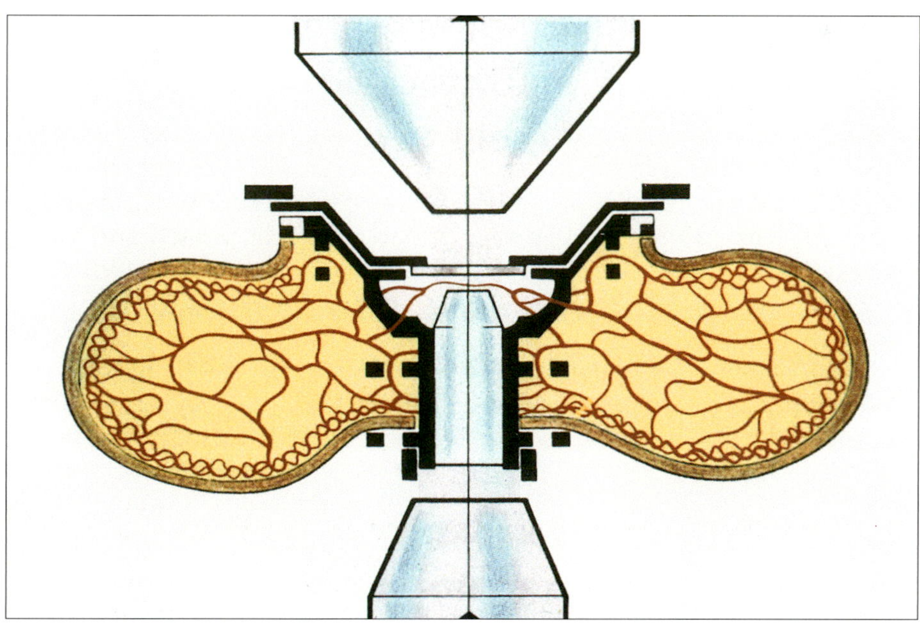

Fig 1-5 Cross section of the titanium chamber with microscope elements installed into a skin tube.

microscope, the tiny balls of fat moving through Lundborg's microcirculation looked like a cloud of mosquitoes.

The action of smoking was shown to have a dramatic effect on the microcirculation. After only a few puffs on a cigarette by a volunteer, considerable changes occurred – body temperature dropped, blood pressure increased, the heart beat more rapidly, and the veins became blocked so blood had to seek new pathways. After 2 years at Gothenburg University studying the effects of smoking, research team member Makishige Asano returned to Japan to continue this work. He has spent much of his working life trying to deter people from smoking because of the damage he can see taking place at the cellular level after only a few puffs on a cigarette.

As well as observing these changes, the team also analyzed the effects of various circulatory and alimentary conditions such as low flow states, stasis, hyperlipemia, and diabetic vasculopathy (Fig 1-6). The results of this research are well documented and also formed the basis of several doctoral theses for Brånemark's student group. The microcirculation laboratory run by Brånemark proved a very fertile place for a huge range of research, and its demand for multidisciplinary skills was a key factor in the ultimate breakthrough in osseointegration.

In essence, the work revealed the dynamic nature of blood. It had a beauty and elegance and a kind of poetry in the way it responded and adapted to changing conditions. Brånemark has famously stated, "As one observes the blood cells at length in the circulation, they acquire a permanent and individual personality."

These sets of experiments on microcirculation were successful in that they revealed the behavior and structure of microcirculation with a clarity that had never been achieved previously. This complemented the work Brånemark had carried out in bone, but it also started the seeds of an idea in his mind. In both cases, titanium components, ie, chambers, had been used to support the observation elements *in vivo*. In both the bone and tissue studies there was no rejection of the metal by the body. In the 1960s, researchers were beginning to look more closely for materials that could be used for a range of implantation purposes. Biocompatible materials were beginning to have a variety of applications – as temporary support during healing of complex fractures, to encapsulate devices such as heart pacemakers, and as hip joint replacements, for example.

There is always a risk, however small, that the body will reject foreign components, leading to inflammation and the need to remove artificial

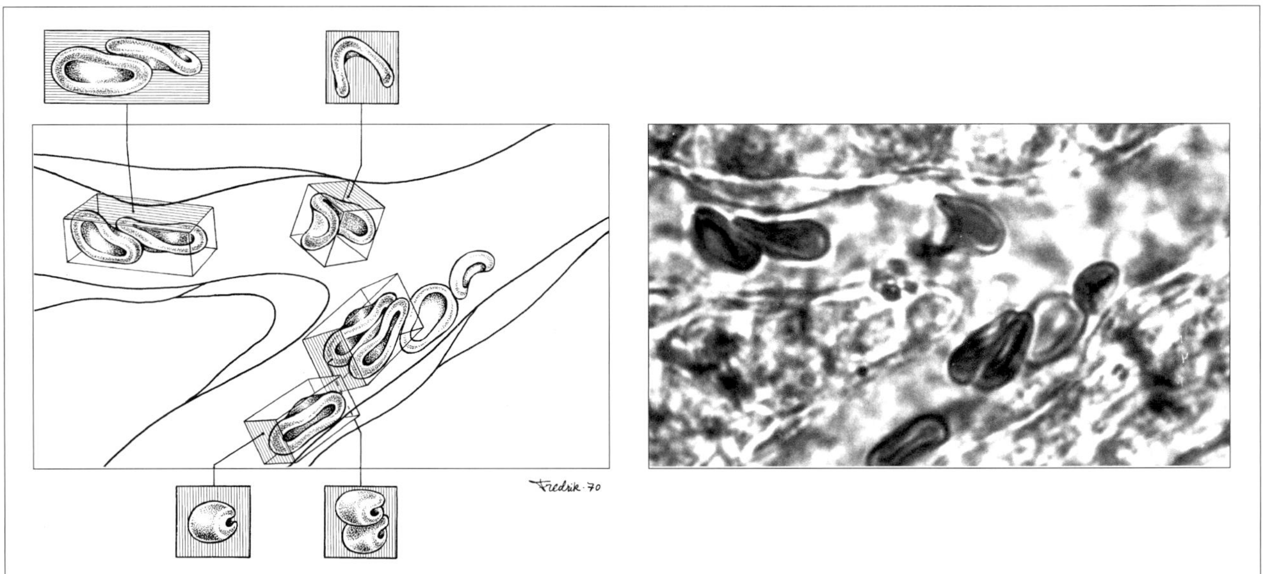

Fig 1-6 Classical illustrations of red blood cells moving through the microcirculation as observed using light microscopy. As the red cells move, they deform, but their basic biconcave shape is always maintained. The study was intended to show what human blood cells look like and how they behave in the nutritive part of circulation under normal flow conditions, during low flow states, and during complete stasis of varying duration.

implants. What surprised Brånemark was that titanium caused no inflammation and that the titanium chambers remained in place for so long without problems. Further, this made him wonder about the potential of titanium to act as an anchorage point for load-bearing medical applications, such as the connection of artificial limbs.

This was the spur to the next set of experiments – to test if titanium could be used as a bridge in bone-healing applications.

Bone-Healing Experiments

At the point at which Brånemark and his colleagues embarked upon further studies, they knew two key things from their previous work with titanium components. First, titanium had the ability to become an integral part of living bone and was accepted by bone as part of its own structure. Second, it was also accepted by soft tissue and did not cause the major inflammation that can lead to rejection. At the time Brånemark was working with titanium, it was not known if other materials showed this peculiar ability to bond with bone (Fig 1-7). Titanium was an exotic material, and little knowledge was available about working with the metal in general industry. Its main use was military, as it is a lightweight and strong metal capable of withstanding high temperatures. In the 1950s, aircraft designers began to incorporate titanium alloys. One of the first uses was in the highly successful Pratt and Whitney J57 engine. Between the years 1947 and 1957, generous funding from the American government resulted in the rapid development of titanium alloy technology. From the 1960s, a gradual reduction in the cost of titanium and its alloys opened up applications in the chemical and medical fields. This is because the thin layer of titanium oxide that encapsulates the pure metal is highly resistant to the most corrosive of materials. It is particularly resistant to attack from highly reactive chlorides such as bleaching agents, hot brine, ferric chloride, and chlorinated hydrocarbons. So, the chemical processing industry quickly found that titanium could be used for piping and tubing applications. The petrochemical industry also adopted titanium in its processing plants.

In reality, the titanium oxide that comes into contact with other substances is the most important aspect of the metal's properties. The basic metal is highly reactive, and this makes it quite a challenge for materials engineers. Fortunately, at the time of Brånemark's studies, engineers were learning techniques that could be applied to work with this material successfully.

As noted, titanium is a difficult metal to make into components because it is soft and can cause damage to cutting tools. Titanium is a relatively poor conductor of heat compared with other metals. A tungsten carbide cutting tool operating at a constant speed would generate a temperature of 700°C working with titanium, but only 540°C when working with steel. Since the heat from the cutting tool does not transfer as easily to titanium as it does to steel, there is a risk that the cutting tool may weld to the titanium workpiece. This highlights the difference in conduction and requires the skills of a fine mechanic with a deep interest in working with difficult materials.

From the time Brånemark moved to Gothenburg, he was able to call upon the talents of Viktor Kuikka. Kuikka was employed at the university to provide mechanical support for those needing special tools and components. Until Brånemark's arrival in Gothenburg, this watchmaker by trade had never found his own considerable skills put to the test. From the moment these two men met – an extroverted professor with ideas and a quiet, practical man who could

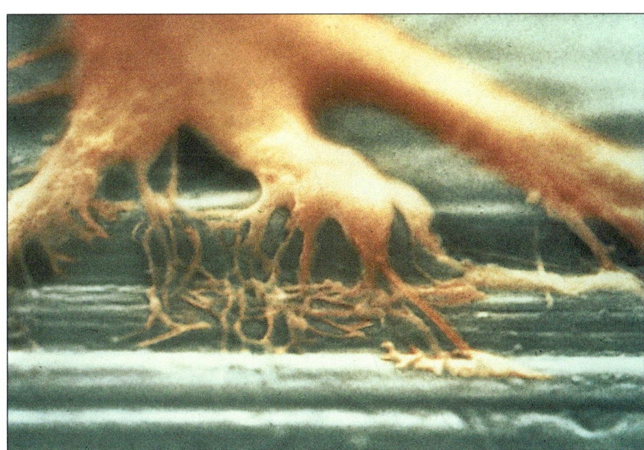

Fig 1-7 A scanning electron micrograph shows clearly how bone cells have made a strong attachment to the titanium surface. This elegantly illustrates that the process of osseointegration has been successful.

nurse any metal into any shape – there was a silent understanding between them. As Brånemark once said, "He did not talk a lot, but he thought a lot."

Kuikka had spent several years working at a telecommunications company prior to joining the university. A refugee from one of the Baltic states, he had spent some years working on entrepreneurial pursuits such as the manufacture of ballpoint pens. However, these ambitions came to nothing and Kuikka settled down to use his skills in the traditional manufacturing industry.

Kuikka made the titanium components for the blood flow studies and willingly moved on to making the titanium parts required for the next series of experiments. Over the years, Kuikka laid the ground rules for the design and manufacture of all the major components and surgical instruments that underpin the osseointegration technique.

Brånemark has always acknowledged Kuikka's contribution to this work. He says Kuikka understood the demands of the medical use of titanium and knew how to produce components to the most stringent standards. Indeed, Kuikka's influence on the mechanical aspects of the work was such that no component or piece of instrumentation produced in the workshop could be used if he did not approve it fit for its purpose. This reliance on Kuikka's skills continued for many years and helped lay the foundation for the commercialization of the technology in the 1980s.

While Kuikka created and produced the basic components, Brånemark and his team moved onto devising the next key set of experiments that would be fundamental to osseointegration. With suggestions from other surgeons, Brånemark had to establish the key factors that would guarantee the best conditions for osseointegration to occur. In essence, these were complete sterility, prevention of contamination, minimal tissue violence, and precision.

Conditions for Osseointegration

Precision is a matter of engineering accuracy. Brånemark felt that all instruments and components used in the osseointegration work should conform to very fine tolerances. This would ensure close congruence between the implant and its bone location for an accurate fit. *Minimal tissue violence* requires a surgical technique that handles both hard and soft tissue very gently. As Brånemark commented, "It is tempting to screw in the fixtures too hard." Inserting fixtures is done with sharp, disposable drills with light and intermittent drilling pressure and the incremental removal of bone using drills of increasing diameters in conjunction with the general application of water irrigation. *Complete sterility* is the normal goal in any operation. *Avoidance of contamination* means ensuring that the titanium components do not touch other metals, rubber gloves, or cotton towels as any chemical elements adhering to these surfaces may result in unfavorable conditions for osseointegration.

These prerequisites for success were based on Brånemark's own observations and, to some extent, feelings. In 1979, Professor Bengt Kasemo and coworkers, including Jukka Lausmaa, at Sweden's Chalmers University of Technology, began a collaboration that confirmed most of these observations. It was important to establish and define "a clean surface." To the eye, a surface may look clean, but it may be chemically contaminated with a number of molecular layers of foreign species. The Chalmers team developed standard methods and routines for analyzing the surface of the titanium and its related oxide. They looked at a large range of materials and technology questions, including how chemical treatments such as cleaning and sterilization during component manufacture might alter or contaminate the titanium oxide surface that protects the bulk titanium. Later this work was key to the development of the sterile packaging used in the commercial production of titanium components.

"Our original idea was to work with knee joint and hip joint surgery, with the victims of motorcycle accidents, but working in the mouth turned out to be much better for the initial clinical experience," recalls Brånemark. It was chance that the first patient considered suitable for the first clinical procedure had dental problems.

The Battle for Approval

"It is the customary fate of new truths to begin as heresies and to end as superstitions."
Thomas Henry Huxley, 1822-1900

Having prepared the groundwork and believing in the research data already gathered, Brånemark and his team at Gothenburg University felt ready to move into clinical trials for their bone-healing techniques. For a number of reasons, not least the existence of real patient need, dentistry was the first clinical application in 1965.

The First Patient

The first patient, Gösta Larsson, had suffered a lifetime of dental problems. He had a cleft palate, a deformed chin and jaw, and had lost the teeth in his lower jaw. At the time, he was 34 years old and experiencing constant pain and discomfort that affected his ability to eat and talk. Because his chin and jaw had been untreatable during his adolescent years, Larsson was resigned to living with these defects for the rest of his life (Fig 2-1).

Larsson described his existence before remedial treatment using osseointegration: "I couldn't even chew a slice of bread. The few teeth I had were, more or less, randomly distributed through my mouth and not where they were supposed to be. My jawbone was not very strong, either. At the time, I was hardly living an ordinary life. I'd grown up with the problem of not being able to chew properly. Although I had learned to cope, not being able to chew and being told that there isn't very much the dentist can do is the kind of thing you accept."

Then, on a visit to his dentist, he was given the news that a novel technique had become available with the potential to improve his situation dramatically. Larsson had no hesitation in offering to participate in clinical trials.

Patients selected for this pioneering work were those for whom conventional treatment was either inappropriate or had failed. Larsson's situation was beyond resolution by conventional treatment possibilities (Fig 2-2). This continued to be the pattern for patient selection throughout the development of treatment regimes using osseointegration.

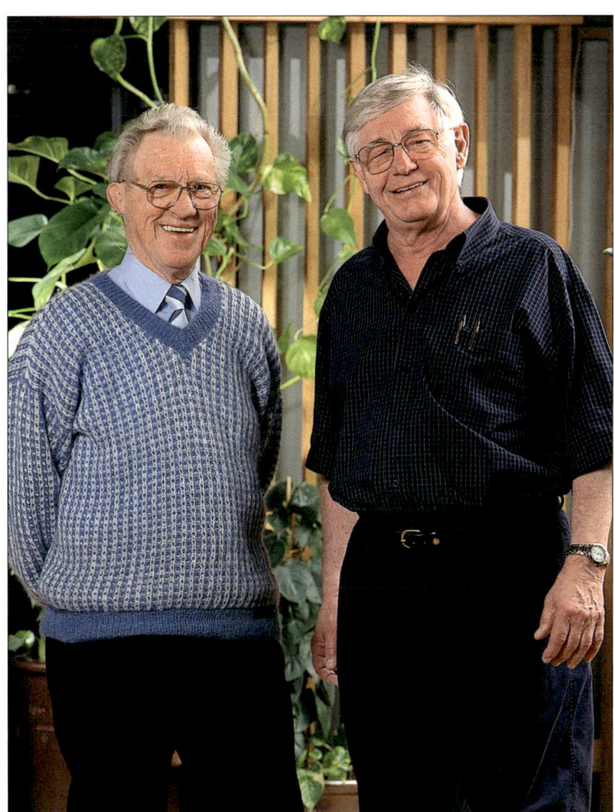

Fig 2-1 Gösta Larsson, pictured at left with Professor Brånemark, was the first person to receive bone-anchored dental implants. Today, those implants are still functioning successfully and he has received further osseointegration treatments, including an attachment for a bone-anchored hearing aid that sits behind his ear.

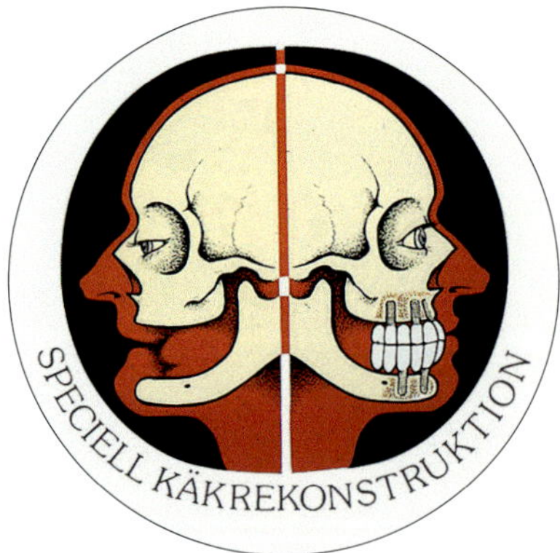

Fig 2-2 Concept for a jawbone-anchored dental prosthesis. Image produced by artist Fredrik Johansson in 1977.

Surgical Procedure

Brånemark and his colleagues, Uno Breine, Olle Hallén (Fig 2-3), and Alf Öhrman (Fig 2-4), had established the basic design of titanium screws with threads to allow in-growth of bone. They developed a surgical technique to ensure minimal tissue injury and required the same care and delicate touch as for the more obviously vulnerable parts of the body. Brånemark had always felt that gentle handling of tissue and bone could promote healing. This view was not shared by many orthopedic surgeons of the time.

To ensure that the surgical procedure could be controlled and monitored precisely, it was carried out in two stages. During the first stage, implants were inserted into bone using a very gentle surgical technique. The first step in this phase of surgery was to drill small holes in the jawbone tissue using relatively low drill speeds plus copious irrigation with saline solution to keep the temperature within established, safe limits. Once the operation site had been prepared, the titanium implant was carefully screwed into place. The amount of pressure applied as the implant was installed was monitored to prevent applying excess force. The site of the operation and the implant were then covered with a permucosal flap and allowed to heal for 3 to 6 months.

To ensure that the implant was undisturbed, patients were asked to avoid using their conventional dentures for a week or two. The idea was to allow the crucial healing phase, in which the bone tissue forms in close apposition to the titanium implant, to be given the best conditions for osseointegration to occur.

Before the second operation, radiographs were taken to ensure that osseointegration had been successful and also to locate each implant. If osseointegration had occurred, the surgeons opened up the site and attached the abutments, or permucosal attachments, which were essentially titanium cylinders that created connection points for any dental prosthesis – a single tooth or a complete set of false teeth. With the abutments in place, and after a few weeks of further

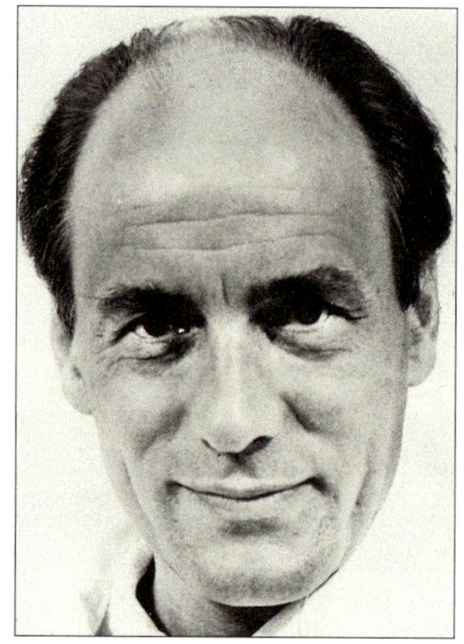

Fig 2-3 Olle Hallén worked closely with Brånemark on developing suitable surgical procedures for the osseointegration technique.

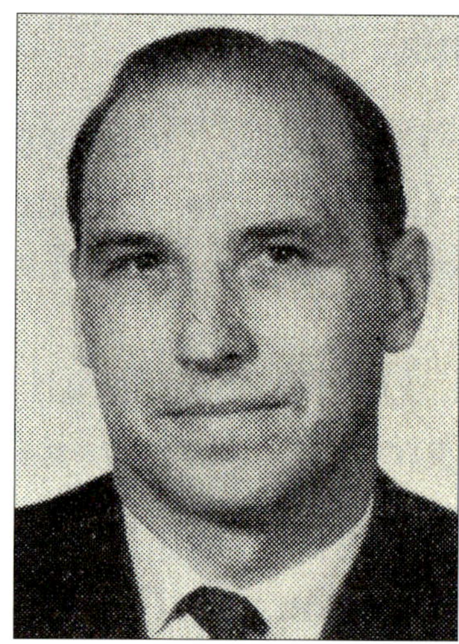

Fig 2-4 Alf Öhrman was a strong supporter of osseointegration and helped devise its dental procedures.

healing, a cast could be made to create the final prosthesis that would be screwed to the abutment.

Here, then, is the original procedure for osseointegration as applied to dentistry, though today it can be carried out in a single step.

The use of this two-stage procedure during early clinical treatment had a key benefit. Should a problem occur at any of the stages, or even after the prosthesis was fixed, the components could be removed, leaving the patient in the same position as before treatment.

Success

For Gösta Larsson, however, this pioneering operation was a success. Though Larsson had a weak jawbone, the team was able to place four implants into the bone. These were used as anchors for a fixed set of dentures. Once the treatment was completed, Larsson recorded a dramatic improvement in his quality of life. The ability to chew and eat food normally resulted in his gaining weight, and apart from his enhanced enjoyment of all things culinary, Larsson found that his speech and appearance also improved. Thirty-five years later, Larsson is still enjoying life with his teeth firmly in place.

Despite the success of this first operation, Brånemark proceeded with extreme caution. In fact, it was more than a year before the team carried out further clinical work on human patients. Brånemark was treading a very thin line professionally. He and his colleagues had always envisioned orthopedic applications, Brånemark's own particular area of interest, as the first to reach clinical reality.

The fact that a dental application presented itself first had both positive and negative effects. From a practical point of view, of all the possible sites in the body to insert titanium implants, the mouth is one of the best for reviewing the success of osseointegration. As Brånemark pointed out, "All the patient has to do is open his or her mouth and you can see what is going on." As clinical trials continued, dental applications provided important information and experience relating to the acceptance of titanium components in both bone and tissue.

Professional Resistance

However, the negative aspects were almost overwhelming at the time. These included the tremendous hostility of the dental community in Sweden to Brånemark's work, not least because Brånemark was not a dental researcher. From the outset, Brånemark had always considered the work on osseointegration to be of a multidisciplinary nature and had collaborated with relevant specialists including dentists, other surgeons, and engineers. Unfortunately, this did not soften or divert criticism. The dislike of an "outsider" manifested itself in a number of ways, at times swinging violently between moments of high drama and comic farce.

One such occasion took place in 1969. Brånemark had been asked to speak to the Swedish dental community in the small, southern town of Landskrona, Sweden. Some of Brånemark's colleagues and doctoral students drove to the hall to watch him deliver this important lecture. Though nervous about delivering his talk to a hall full of dentists and academics, he gave his speech in his usual high-speed and lively manner. The audience response to his information bemused his loyal students. In essence, the natives were hostile.

One famous and well-respected Swedish dental professor, Hilding Björn, could not contain his anger at Brånemark's impudence in carrying out research in a field for which he had not trained. He rose from his seat and commented that he could not rely on the information he had just heard, exclaiming, "I do not trust people who publish themselves in the *Readers' Digest*!" This was a reference to an article published about Brånemark's earlier work on microcirculation. Many academics, at that time, considered having research published outside learned scientific journals a poor reflection on the reputation of the researcher. However, the article relating to the microcirculation work was, in fact, written by an independent writer, not Brånemark himself. This in some ways negated the criticism but did not prevent it.

Brånemark, however, could not resist the verbal counterattack. Björn had supported a leading brand of tooth products. His name was printed on each packet, which prompted the retort by Brånemark: "I don't trust people who publish themselves on the back of a toothpick." The war of words then escalated as another member of the audience joined in shouting, "Sir, you are a humbug. You are not even a dentist!" Brånemark was not silenced by that remark, either. "It is true that I am not a dentist, but I am happy to train them," he replied. As Associate Professor of Anatomy at Gothenburg University, Brånemark frequently gave lectures and examinations to dental students.

This was just the first incident of many Brånemark encountered. It set the trend for at least a decade. If any of Brånemark's students attending the lecture had believed the academic world was one in which gentile behavior was the norm, they were disabused of that belief. The personal and professional attacks took a variety of forms and Brånemark, with his work providing him a strong professional platform, was determined to stand his ground. As he freely admits, tact is not a commodity in which he is overly endowed. "If I were in the diplomatic business," he says wryly, "there would be a new war every day." This adversarial nature, however, proved important to the future acceptance of osseointegration. It is fortunate that such criticism, or the other challenges he would face, in bringing osseointegration to clinical reality during those early years had not cowed Brånemark. As former student, Björn Rydevik, now an eminent professor, noted, "For a period of 10 years, it appeared that Brånemark's struggles were uphill against a strong headwind."

There were a number of other curious developments, including the attempt to denigrate Brånemark's work through the circulation of an audiotape attacking the man and his discovery. Though this could be regarded as a very infantile attack, much enjoyed by Brånemark's students during break times, it was a symptom of deeper troubles ahead.

On November 15, 1973, the National Odontological Assembly, one of Sweden's leading dental associations, discussed Brånemark's work at a meeting in Stockholm. The "Gothenburg method" was condemned, with one newspaper stating that the assembly was "negatively disposed" to it. Comments made at this gathering included the belief that as the dental implant perforated the mucous membrane it "destroyed the

mouth's protection against infection." The method was variously labeled dangerous, expensive, and painful with patients likely to regret their "fixed teeth" as a costly mistake.

The proceedings then began to indulge in personal attacks on Brånemark, who was not there to defend himself. Though the chairman of the meeting did not appear to prevent such remarks, they did cause offense to one of the participants, Alf Öhrman, a deeply respected member of the academic dental fraternity and a board member of the Swedish Dental Academy. At the time, he was chief surgeon and head of the department of oral diagnostics at the odontology clinic in Gothenburg. Importantly, he knew Brånemark personally and had worked with him professionally. He was so outraged by the behavior at this meeting that he threatened to resign from this august academic body if the assembly did not apologize to Brånemark. A few weeks after the meeting, Brånemark received a letter of apology, but attacks on his osseointegration work continued for at least another 5 years in various forms.

While it may be difficult to understand the need for personal attacks on a medical researcher, there were some valid foundations for concerns related to implant technology. The whole perception of dental implants at that time had been as a failed and dangerous technology. Even Brånemark, then and now, avoids the use of the word "implant" in his work because of the history of dental implants that preceded his own developments. So bad was the reputation of earlier work that the dental community had universally condemned its clinical use. In the United States it was even considered unacceptable human experimentation because some implant designs left patients in a far worse state than prior to their treatment.

From the outset of his research into the clinical applications of osseointegration, Brånemark had set a clear goal. The titanium implants or components were carefully designed so if they failed and had to be removed, the patient would not be left in a worse state than before the treatment. Brånemark had also felt the technology and techniques being evolved through osseointegration should be capable of being adapted or superceded should better treatment regimes become available. The light of experience has led Brånemark to modify his own approach to osseointegration when clinical and other research highlights better ways of doing things. He points out that assumptions should always be challenged and the evidence of clinical experience should be used to help improve and refine techniques.

Brånemark has always been meticulous in his documentation of clinical and research results. This has proved itself time and time again, especially during those crucial moments when osseointegration was being evaluated by the medical establishment. On a number of occasions osseointegration came under extremely close scrutiny, and Brånemark was faced with battling against the might of bureaucracy and the distrust of fellow academics.

At the outset of early trials into implanted devices, this attention to detail, coupled with the need to gather reliable long-term data, had brought Brånemark into conflict with government-funding authorities. There are a number of key moments when the entire body of research was under threat, but Brånemark stood his ground.

One of the most serious clashes with "the powers that be" was following the early animal studies carried out in the 1960s. Having completed the studies, Brånemark felt that it was important to the research that the harrier dogs used in the experiments be allowed to live out their natural lives. Regular checks to see that the implants were functioning well over the long term was providing valuable data for the osseointegration team. The longer the animals lived, the more information was available about the stability of fixtures. Many of the dogs lived 7 or more years. The first experimental animal was an old dog called Onclas who had outlived his usefulness as a hunting dog. Instead of being destroyed, he was donated to the clinic and became a much-loved pet who lived a further 10 years and helped the team learn much about osseointegration.

In many ways, the dogs were considered part of the team. They all had names and were regularly exercised and visited. One of the vets became so fond of one of the dogs that she took him home on weekends and gave him a permanent home once the studies had been concluded. So when the medical body funding these studies, the Swedish Medical Research Council, instructed Brånemark to destroy the dogs, he was horrified and refused. As well as destroying perfectly healthy animals that were loved and well cared for, "killing the dogs would have meant losing valuable long-term data and would also destroy a great deal of the research already carried out," explained Brånemark.

This issue soured the relationship between Brånemark and the research council for years. The discussions reached a stalemate and some of Brånemark's colleagues urged him to give in and comply with the council's requests. However, despite the weight of the opposition, he managed to win the argument, even if he lost some friends as a result. Without Brånemark's commitment and belief in the work, osseointegration would have faltered in the face of many hurdles. Tomas Albrektsson, now professor of handicap research at Gothenburg University, was a student of Brånemark's during those turbulent years. Of Brånemark, Albrektsson admitted, "If he hadn't been a dominant kind of person, there would be no oral implants today."

Private Practice

In terms of resolve in the face of difficulty, 1968 was a crucial year. Brånemark and his team found themselves cut off from the support of the local hospital system and the university facilities because of the worsening relationships between the research body and Brånemark. Gösta Larsson and a few other early patients were treated at the local Sahlgren's Hospital in Gothenburg, but with a couple of years' encouraging results behind them, Brånemark and his team were faced with having to halt further clinical work. Rather than delay offering treatment to more patients, a private clinic was set up and equipped thanks to 250,000 Swedish crowns borrowed from a local bank. Funds to support the treatment of patients came from a variety of sources – private donations, loans, Swedish industry, charity, and even contributions from patients themselves. Brånemark felt it was important to ensure that the total treatment costs for the patient were within reasonable limits.

The clinic was completely outside the Swedish health insurance system and so overcame the immediate problem of dealing with intran-

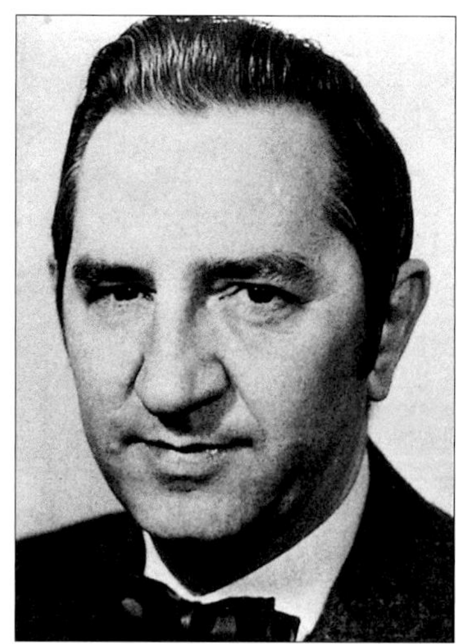

Fig 2-5 Richard Skalak worked with Brånemark from the late 1960s and was an outside observer to the challenges met during the development of osseointegration. Skalak remained on the board of the Institute for Applied Biotechnology as its chairman until his death in 1997 at the age of 74.

sigent institutions. It also helped with the assessment of the type of health care resources that would be required once the technique was accepted by the national health system. The clinic also provided the appropriate clinical data to be presented to the health authorities. Brånemark and the team still had the goal of making osseointegration an accepted part of dental treatment in suitable and carefully selected cases. He believed strongly in a cost benefit to be gained by treating certain types of patients. Often patients with severe dental conditions present with other medical problems such as depression, which can be a considerable financial cost to the health care system. Brånemark argued that the initial high cost of treatment with osseointegration was more than offset by the positive effects on patients' overall health and the resulting long-term savings in medical care.

Despite this exclusion of the clinic from national health care, there was a certain measure of support for osseointegration and sympathy for Brånemark's desire to help patients. The local health authority, in the form of the hospital management in Gothenburg, looked at a variety of options to alleviate the clinic's lack of funding. This action was taken because of the support of Thure Höglund, director of the Gothenburg health care system, who had seen the effectiveness of osseointegration first hand,

and his colleague, Olle Holmstrand. Initially the lack of clinical data, coupled with difficulties in integrating the work within the prevailing medical and dental health care system, made it impossible for the treatment to gain formal adoption. Gradually both problems were solved.

The Gothenburg Hospital Authority managed to provide some financial support, having made the decision that "not economic but medical and odontological factors should decide whether a person should be able to undergo oral rehabilitation." The National Social Welfare Board, which was the ultimate funding body, did not react negatively to this statement. As a result, some financial resources came from the state though the clinic still had to run on a very limited budget. Richard Skalak, a biomechanics researcher from the United States and one of Brånemark's close colleagues (Fig 2-5), commented, "I believe that there was a time that, without official approval, Brånemark carried on the pilot studies using his own personal funds."

What had been conceived, as a temporary measure, while the authorities deliberated on the acceptance of osseointegration, ended up lasting 6 years, during which 233 patients were treated. The clinic continued to work closely with the ear, nose, and throat (ENT) and plastic surgery clinics at Sahlgren's Hospital and the odontological clinic in Gothenburg. This helped to accumulate independent data and follow-up information crucial to providing the evidence for osseointegration.

Richard Skalak, who visited frequently during these years, noted, "During the 1970s, there were alternative periods of success and gloom. The clinical experiences and results were mostly favorable. The gloom and difficulties seemed to stem mostly from the difficulty of persuading the dental community that the method worked and should be supported" by the Swedish national or local health systems.

There were a number of occasions when Brånemark reflected on the wisdom of battling against the odds. "Sometimes, I felt that it would have been rational to do something else," he has admitted. However, there were a number of key individuals whose professional and personal support were crucial in maintaining the momentum. Olle Hallén, according to Skalak, was "a strong, impartial, and influential supporter of

Brånemark's methods, to have the technique officially recognized and approved."

Hallén, who died in 1990, was also a gifted surgeon. He worked within the ENT department of Sahlgren's Hospital and collaborated with Brånemark on many of the surgical techniques as they apply to osseointegration. Brånemark has always gratefully acknowledged this man's contribution to the successful clinical application of osseointegration. When Brånemark set up the Institute for Applied Biotechnology in 1978 to further research and collaboration in osseointegration, Hallén was asked to be chairman of the board. He occupied this position until 1985, when ill health forced him to resign. Others who have occupied this position are Kåre Larsson, Sven Malmström, and Skalak.

National Examination and Approval

It was the sustained and strong support of colleagues such as Hallén and Skalak, who continued to visit with suggestions for testing the mechanical aspects of osseointegration, that helped to affirm Brånemark's own determination to keep the work going. Finally, the situation came to a head when the health authority called an independent panel to assess the osseointegration work. This was an unusual step on behalf of the authorities as such panels are rarely convened. Many colleagues were convinced that the dental community, still suspicious of Brånemark's work, hoped that this would reveal osseointegration as an elaborate hoax. Tomas Albrektsson commented, "This panel was the kind normally set up to deal with quacks."

Whatever the motivation, this panel was to settle the issue of osseointegration within Sweden. On two consecutive days, February 18 and 19, 1975, three professors from Umeå University in the north of Sweden, Axel Bergenholtz, Bo Bergman, and Max Lundberg, carried out their scrutiny of Brånemark's work. At random, 20 patients treated in Gothenburg were chosen from the 165 people who had received fixtures since 1965. Seventeen of them were able to attend the clinic for the Umeå professors' assessment of their dental state. As well as examining patients, the visiting team looked at the fixtures, the construction and fitting of the dental bridges, and radiographic information.

The nature of the Swedish health care system, coupled with the fact that Brånemark has always been meticulous in the follow-up and care of individual patients, yielded a wealth of information about how patients were treated and the success of the procedure. All the data the scrutinizing team required were readily available. Having studied this information, they departed to prepare their report to the National Health and Welfare Board.

Three agonizing months were to pass before the report was officially published. On May 22, 1975, Brånemark and his team received a copy of the report. It was a document read from cover to cover! Brånemark commented that the report had turned osseointegration from an experimental technique to "lege artis." The key conclusions of the report were that the implants worked and were stable. In it, the three professors stated that "treatment with a jaw-bone-anchored bridge construction can and should be used as a complement to conventional prosthetics."

The professors did feel the use of titanium implants should be a last resort. They explained in the report, "One of the main indications should be that conventional prosthetic methods have been tried and, for different reasons, failed." Three basic criteria were set by the panel for the selection and treatment of patients with the osseointegration technique. They covered factors such as mouth hygiene instruction for patients and preoperative analysis and construction of the dental bridges, as well as suggesting some improvements to the overall esthetic results.

On October 10, 1975, the official letter came from the National Health and Welfare Board stating that the implant method developed by Brånemark should be considered a bona fide treatment. It reiterated the scrutinizing team's opinion that it was a treatment of last resort and added that the treatment should be carried out by properly trained specialists at a suitably resourced center.

For Brånemark and the team, this letter marked the end of working outside the country's national health service. Six months later on April 1, 1976, the clinic was fully incorporated into the National Insurance System, and the Hospital Authority in Gothenburg brought the Brånemark method into its scheme on May 11, 1976. Funding for osseointegration was now available from the Hospital Authority, and the treatment could be offered within the state health care system from June 1 of that year.

Crucially, funding was made available for a dedicated unit for jaw construction at the odontological clinic in Gothenburg. Ulf Lekholm, one of Brånemark's early collaborators, headed this unit. Dubbed the Brånemark Clinic, it was set up in 1986 and still operates under that name today.

By July 1976, the funding situation was eased to such an extent that Brånemark was able to transfer the private work carried at a clinic in the Gothenburg suburb of Mölndal to the dental school in Gothenburg. It was to become the first center of expertise in dental applications for osseointegration, as the scrutinizing professors had been convinced this was a technique outside the capabilities of the general dentist. They believed that specialist teams with considerable resources – surgical expertise, radiographic diagnostics, prosthetic technicians, and peridontology – should be set up in a limited number of centers throughout Sweden.

Indeed, the state health authority was now willing to provide funds for such centers, and in October 1977, the first course on oral rehabilitation incorporating osseointegrated fixtures was held. Brånemark personally ran the course, to which some of Sweden's most respected dental experts were invited.

The Spread of Knowledge

All the early courses in oral rehabilitation were supervised personally by Brånemark. He was trying to ensure that, from the outset, the osseointegration technique would be based on the very careful surgical procedures that had been painstakingly evolved. Having faced heavy criticism and fierce opposition to his work, he now wanted to ensure that his good clinical results were not put into jeopardy through misapplication of osseointegration or inadequately trained practitioners.

For the next few years, Brånemark concentrated on training specialists and refining the im-

plants and related components and equipment so knowledge could be transferred into the industry or put on a more commercial footing.

The demand for training and requests for information were encouraging, but also exhausting. Brånemark wanted to ensure that future clinicians working with osseointegration not only had the right tools for the job but also the right attitude and philosophy.

Unlike other procedures, osseointegration implies a team approach, and this collaborative way of working has to be carefully nurtured. Brånemark would only train those he felt could take to heart the gentle nature of the surgery and the need to communicate with other professionals and the patient and who would focus on keeping the patient at the center of care.

Gradually, the training in Sweden was established and Brånemark had to face another major decision. It was time to spread the information to other countries. Even though there was growing acceptance of osseointegration in Sweden, Brånemark was, naturally, hesitant to present his work to an international audience. There were a number of occasions when he turned away from opportunities that presented themselves, to the frustration of his colleagues.

Brånemark was not without international contacts, however. One important figure in that regard was Professor George Zarb of the Faculty of Dentistry at Toronto University in Canada. Zarb was considered one of the leaders in his research field and was much respected by his peers. In the early 1970s, he had read Brånemark's research on dogs, which had been carried out in the mid-1960s. At the time, Zarb was pursuing the possibilities of developing artificial replacements for tooth roots. The possibilities of osseointegration in this regard were clear.

Contact between the two professors was established through a third person, Professor Gunnar E. Carlsson, an eminent prosthodontist. In 1975, Zarb visited Brånemark in Gothenburg and was immediately fascinated and impressed. At one point, Zarb spent 6 months in Sweden to learn the details of Brånemark's work. During that time he persuaded Brånemark to invite researchers from other parts of the world to carry out replication studies.

Zarb returned to Canada, and his group became the first team outside Sweden to participate in parallel studies. These studies confirmed the results that Brånemark's team, and by now others in Sweden, had been achieving for some time. Patrik Henry, working at the Royal Perth Hospital in Australia, also participated in parallel studies. Henry received training in osseointegration methods in 1980. He also confirmed the excellent results in clinical trials that Brånemark achieved in Gothenburg. As the overseas teams had replicated the high survival rates of dental implants in bone, Brånemark's colleagues urged him to go international.

Contacts were made in Japan, too. This came about through the auspices of Professor Gunnar Hambraeus, who promoted scientific collaboration between Sweden and Japan, and the Swedish Ambassador to Japan at that time, Gunnar Lonaeus.

During meetings of the board of the Institute of Applied Biotechnology, which were organized to further research and development of osseointegration, a presentation of the work at an international conference was deemed appropriate. As Skalak recalled, "Brånemark was somewhat leery of setting up this conference but thought the strategy of asking the American university community to take the lead in introducing the new method was a good idea. It turned out to be a proper and successful route."

The Toronto Conference

To smooth the introduction of osseointegration outside Sweden, George Zarb not only offered to provide his academic support but also to carry out much of the organization of the conference, which would take place in Canada in May 1982 at the Four Seasons Hotel in Toronto. Entitled "Osseointegration in Clinical Dentistry," the conference was supported financially by the universities of Toronto and Gothenburg and through grants awarded by the Ministry of Health of Ontario in Canada, plus some industrial funding.

Zarb took the unusual step of writing personal letters to leading researchers in dentistry urging them not to miss the opportunity to learn something new. Skalak noted that the majority of those attending the conference had been drawn by Zarb's reputation alone. Many of those attending said later that they had been curious but had few expectations that implant technology would be any more promising than other systems developed in the past.

Skalak had worked with Brånemark on the early development of the mechanical systems and understood this reaction. Skalak had had conversations with eminent dentists in the United States about the Gothenburg work. "I recall several occasions on which otherwise sound and knowledgeable practitioners and professors in the dental field assured me that there must be some flaw or misunderstanding in the Brånemark system because it was well-known that dental implants simply don't work in the long range," he said. "They, frankly, implied that the reports were too good to be true. I think this is fair index of the revolutionary nature of Brånemark's accomplishments."

As the conference drew close, Brånemark became more apprehensive about the reception he might get. He discussed whether the conference should be delayed so more scientific data could be presented. Colleagues urged him not to falter at this hurdle. They believed 15 years of clinical data, coupled with the international studies, should be convincing enough for even the most skeptical audience. Uncharacteristically, when Brånemark arrived for the Toronto conference he was rather distraught, no doubt contemplating how to defend himself against the might of the international dental community.

Zarb had no such reservations, even though he was taking something of a professional risk in associating himself with a class of treatment still regarded with some skepticism. In the end, the conference was a triumph. Zarb's support turned out to be a crucial factor. He clearly stated his opinion on osseointegration: "The only clinical implant study that has survived scientific scrutiny is the work of Brånemark and his team in Gothenburg, Sweden."

By the end of the conference, the tide of opinion relating to Brånemark's work had turned to such an extent that he was greeted with rapturous applause every time he rose to address the conference.

Some of the researchers attending the conference became close colleagues of Brånemark, striking up relationships that have endured through the years. One of them is Richard Johns, now retired but previously emeritus professor of restorative dentistry at Sheffield University. Johns had good reason to be highly critical of all so-called implant technologies. His doctoral thesis, "A study of the response of tissue to endodontic and endosseous implants in Macaca irus monkeys," completed at London University in 1973, had provided evidence that the implants he investigated were failures in the long term. Johns admits he attended the conference with a very biased view of Brånemark's work. He had no reason to believe osseointegration would produce any better performance than the implants he had studied.

Since that time, Johns has become a very trusted member of Brånemark's circle, occupying a position on the Institute of Applied Biotechnology's Advisory Board. While professor of restorative dentistry at the Charles Clifford Dental Hospital, University of Sheffield, he was responsible for initiating a training center for osseointegration. Johns also organized the first osseointegration course in the United Kingdom in 1987. Though retired, Johns continues to provide his active support, particularly through his involvement in the United Kingdom.

Likewise, David Harris of the Blackrock Clinic in Ireland came to the Toronto conference out of curiosity rather than hope that osseointegration was different from other implant technologies. "I didn't believe it," he said. "We had looked at a variety of implant possibilities. They were very poor and unpredictable and, if they failed, would leave a patient with scarring and bone loss. But the fact that there had been a replicated study in Toronto and the 15 years' study from Brånemark was at total variance with what had gone before."

Also as a result of the Toronto conference, Professor Daniel van Steenberghe, now head of the Laboratory of Oral Physiology at the Catholic University's Leuven's Faculty of Medicine and an internationally renowned researcher and lecturer, started a long collaboration with Brånemark after learning about the technique.

Osseointegration's International Expansion

At this point, one could say "and the rest is history." Life, however, is never that straightfor-

ward. Brånemark returned from his triumph in Canada to a barrage of requests for more information, and he continued to give lectures and run training courses. He had been pre-warned that the response might be enormous. A stockpile of fixtures and other equipment had been built up to anticipate this interest. Despite this, demand was underestimated by a factor of two.

There were a number of key institutions that joined the work in osseointegration. One important center was the Mayo Clinic and Mayo Medical School in the United States. In April 1983, researchers from the Mayo Clinic came to Gothenburg for training. Later that year Brånemark traveled to the United States and participated in the treatment of five carefully selected patients. The Mayo Clinic quickly established a close working relationship with Gothenburg. In that year it became one of five academic institutions in North America to act as training centers for osseointegration.

Today, international collaboration, cooperation, and the sharing of ideas and experience continues at a number of levels. With the platform of the Brånemark Osseointegration Center in Gothenburg as the hub, there is now an international network of clinics with considerable expertise in osseointegration. Gradually, the contact with other specialists, particularly from the Toronto conference, has allowed this collaboration to flourish. There are a number of clinics located in different parts of the world including Boston, Massachusetts, and Spokane and Seattle, Washington, in the United States; Toronto, Canada; Perth, Australia; Leuven, Belgium; and Borås and Malmö, Sweden.

These clinics are complemented by a number of designated Associated Brånemark Osseointegration Centers, which are led by experts in the field of oral and maxillofacial reconstruction and are based in Barcelona and Madrid in Spain; Bauru and São Paulo in Brazil, and Santiago, Chile in South America; Treviso in Italy; Edmonton in Canada; Seoul in Korea; and Tokyo in Japan. The collaboration between these centers is wide-ranging and has always been considered a key resource for the maintenance of high standards in patient care and professional training, as well as contributing to the body of knowledge about osseointegration in general (Fig 2-6).

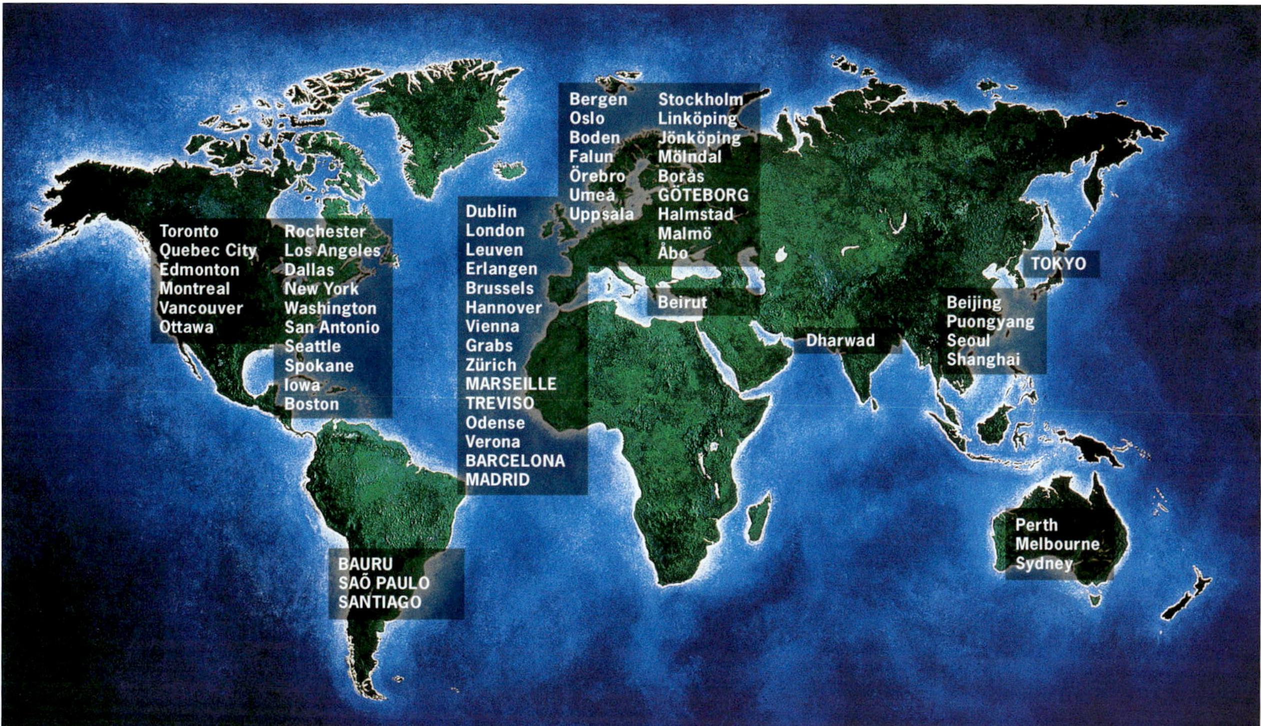

Fig 2-6 Brånemark's work has spread throughout the world with many international centers collaborating on the further development of osseointegration.

It is because of the attention to training, research, and clinical studies that osseointegration has now become an accepted part of the treatment regime in many countries worldwide. It is no longer regarded as the last resort treatment when all else has failed but is often the treatment of choice for those patients or health care systems that have the financial resources to pay for it.

3 On a Sound Footing

"It takes two to speak the truth, one to speak and another to hear."
Henry David Thoreau, 1817-1867

By the time Per-Ingvar Brånemark was ready to demonstrate the success of osseointegration to the world dental community, there was a pressing need to bring the production of the needed surgical components to a more professional level. The small workshop facility in Sweden under the direction of Viktor Kuikka (then the only producer of such osseointegration materials) was already under pressure with requests from Swedish clinicians and already hard pressed to fulfill their component and equipment needs.

As Brånemark had always had a keen interest in engineering and had the undoubted talents of Kuikka on hand, he knew what procedures were necessary to create the right components for osseointegration. Kuikka was more than a technician, and his abilities in fine mechanics were highly respected by Brånemark. Kuikka made significant contributions to the development of all the practical methods by which the osseointegrative screws and instruments were

manufactured (and therefore to the success of the early trials). In a workshop environment, it was relatively straightforward to produce the small quantities of the components, but by the end of the 1970s, it was clear that the implant system needed to be commercialized as demand for dental patient treatment grew.

From the outset, Brånemark had realized the time would come when osseointegration needed commercial input. He had started the search for a suitable industrial partner and began negotiations with a number of companies in the late 1970s. He had hoped to forge a strong and supportive partnership based on mutual respect and with the central aim of serving the patient (Fig 3-1). This ideal partner would prove difficult to find because the competitive nature of the marketplace frequently means business interests are at odds with clinical needs.

Brånemark felt, and still feels, it was important to continually question the motives of commercial interests and sometimes felt he was waging a personal war against adverse business forces and questionable ethics that threaten the quality of treatment for the individual patient. As he had already battled to have the technique accepted clinically, Brånemark believed it was important to set the highest standards for its components and practice. He called on Ove Brandes, an expert in law and business who became involved with attempts to organize the relationship with industry so hardware could be produced for the clinical market.

The work of Uno Zacharisson was also crucial in creating a reliable follow-up regime for each patient that could also generate accurate statistics to measure the effectiveness of osseointegration. Zacharisson and his co-worker, Lars

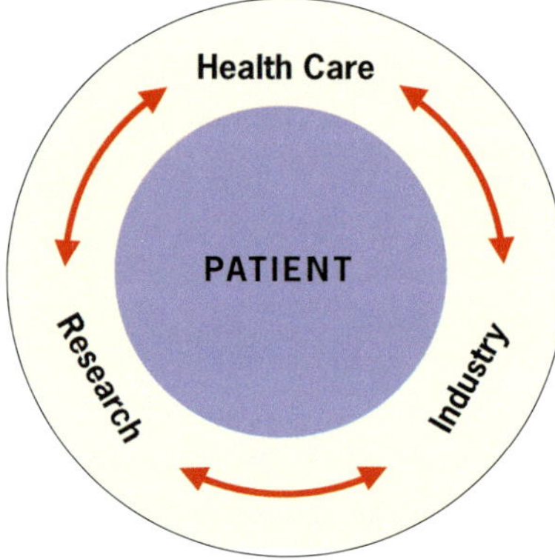

Fig 3-1 This illustration was created to remind those involved in osseointegration of the interplay between each party and their responsibilities to the patient.

Pettersson, enabled Brånemark to analyze large patient groups over decades and to critically scrutinize facts and factors relating to osseointegration. This follow-up system provided, and still provides, a sound platform to follow the clinical work.

That said, Brånemark does not deny that the progress and acceptance of osseointegration was dependent on commercialization with a suitable industrial partner. The spread of treatment relied then, and still relies, heavily on the support of a healthy, profitable, and responsive commercial enterprise with the range of manufacturing and production skills needed to make high-quality components.

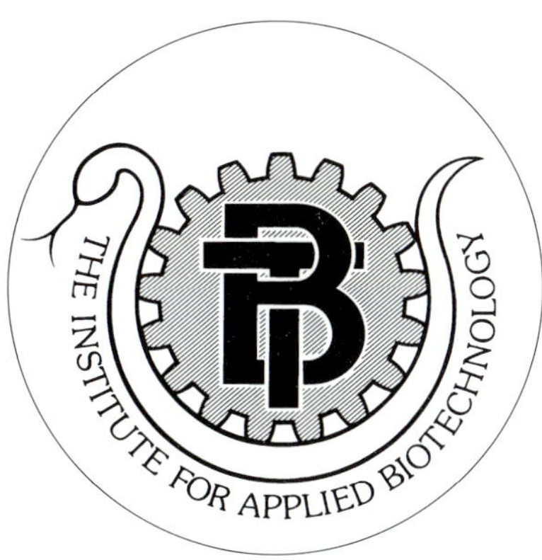

Fig 3-2 The Institute for Applied Biotechnology was set up as a forum for sharing knowledge about the osseointegration technique. Its goal remains that of cooperation and collaboration at the multidisciplinary level.

The Institute for Applied Biotechnology

In 1978, Brånemark set up the Institute for Applied Biotechnology (Fig 3-2). The Institute was intended to be outside the influence of the Swedish State University system, and its aim was to concentrate on the future development of osseointegration in all its forms, as well as to form close ties with academics working in other research fields and with industry. The Institute provided an important forum for discussion between parties whose views were diverse. This included initiating a dialogue with commercial interests.

The Institute's initial board consisted of four of Brånemark's most trusted co-workers. The chairman was Olle Hallén, who had been a trusted supporter even during those difficult times when it appeared other close allies had deserted Brånemark. Brånemark has always had high praise for this very civilized and trustworthy person in whom people tended to confide when they had a problem.

Olle Hallén

Hallén was a very active chairman and promoted the Institute's aims and goals. He was keen to encourage researchers and establish a mechanism by which such workers could gain both recognition and more material rewards for their contributions to osseointegration. While Hallén was chairman, there were many lively debates. In addition, he was a talented surgeon and proposed and developed many practical clinical aspects of the osseointegration work.

Because of his belief in, and commitment to, the osseointegration work, Hallén spoke openly in favor of the technology and in support of its cause. On March 8, 1985, Hallén attended a symposium in Gothenburg and explained some of the immense hurdles to be overcome for any new treatment to be accepted within a national health care system. He used the opportunity to analyze and criticize the way research in Sweden was funded, administered, judged, and, frequently, blocked. Later the government-owned organization, The Technical Development Board, published a document called "Everyone Needs Repair" in which Hallén summarized his perspectives on the issue.

The article highlighted the fact that scientific endeavor has to survive political machinations in the funding system and overcome many layers of bureaucracy that appear designed to stifle the innovative process at the embryonic stage. Hallén said that it was "manifestly difficult for new ideas to thread their way through the crushing machinery of negotiations, budgets, and long-term plans." He pointed out that the competition for research grants was stiff and that science is expensive to fund. "The scarcity of grants had led to increased bureaucracy in the research environment. Behind this lies a legitimate desire to use the money as effectively as possible. At the same time it becomes more difficult to break through with new ideas." Brånemark, always in need of funds for his wide-ranging research, sought grants outside Sweden, frequently finding success with overseas bodies such as the National Institutes of Health in the United States.

Further Hallén noted that osseointegration research had gotten through this highly complex and frustrating system only because of the personality of Per-Ingvar Brånemark. Hallén said that aside from Brånemark's creative talent, he possessed an "extraordinary enthusiasm and stubbornness." He also made mention of the various crises experienced through the years as osseointegration struggled to become accepted.

One of the ways Brånemark was able to break free from the shackles imposed by his own governmental research was to set up the Institute. Hallén said, "Interdisciplinary research in the setting of a free-standing institute gives greater freedom than the university's line organization." Unfortunately, Hallén had to retire from the Institute board in 1985 because of ill health and, sadly, he died 5 years later. However, by that time he could see the osseointegration process well on its way to commercial and clinical success.

Richard Skalak

Also on the board from the Institute's beginning was Richard Skalak. He had begun his collaboration with Brånemark in 1968, when he spent a sabbatical year working in Gothenburg. Skalak remained on the board, succeeding Hallén as its chairman in 1985, until his death in 1997, at age 74. Skalak is a deeply missed colleague; his gentle humor, wisdom, and tremendous insights were huge assets to the osseointegration process. He is remembered as a generous man, willing to share his knowledge with others, and he was an inspirational teacher, always curious to explore new areas.

It was this curiosity that led Skalak to an interest in the young field of biomedical engineering in the 1960s. Skalak is acknowledged as one of the pioneers in this field, mainly because of his contribution to biomechanics research. Skalak worked with many of Brånemark's students, who became professors in their own right. Björn Rydevik is such an example. Rydevik has

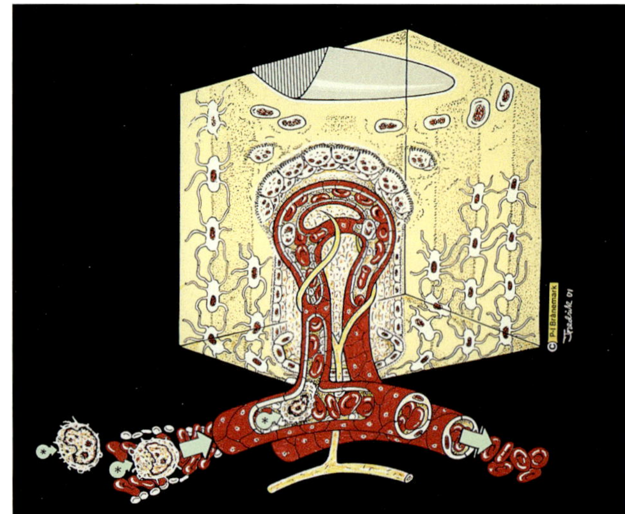

Fig 3-3 Osseointegration, as Skalak understood it, involves biological engineering, supported by microvascular rheology, participating stem cells, and canalicular hydrodynamics.

been awarded a major academic prize in his field of orthopedics. However, he attributes much of his professional success to the fact that he was able to work with Skalak. "He was a fine mentor," commented Rydevik. "I owe him the deepest gratitude for his support." Skalak worked on a huge range of research areas in the biomedical field, including red blood cell rheology, pulmonary circulation, leukocyte function, bone and soft tissue growth, and cell adhesion (Fig 3-3).

As well as bringing his own considerable expertise to osseointegration, Skalak was able to introduce Brånemark and his colleagues to other eminent researchers in a range of disciplines. Over the years, the majority of these people have contributed, and continue to contribute, greatly to the general body of knowledge about osseointegration. Skalak traveled widely throughout the world and published many papers outside his native United States.

Because of his location in the United States, first at Colombia University in New York City and then at the University of California, San Diego after 1988, Skalak could observe the tide of affairs in Sweden from a safe distance. He noted that during the 1970s, "there were alternative periods of success and gloom. The clinical experiences and results were mostly favorable. The gloom and difficulties seemed to stem mostly from the difficulty of convincing the dental community that the method worked and should be supported."

Skalak could see that Brånemark was under enormous pressure at that time. He was not only trying to get the highly skeptical dental fraternity to consider osseointegration as a valid treatment alternative, but funding was also a problem. Brånemark had to carry out a delicate balancing act: juggling finances and spreading whatever monies arrived as widely as possible.

Expansion of Osseointegration

Fortunately, many of these financial concerns were resolved rather quickly once osseointegration became an accepted practice following the official report on the technique. And as mentioned previously, by the end of the 1970s, there was a growing need for a steady flow of existing osseointegration components. There was also a call for new types of components for the growing number of other applications being researched by Brånemark and his colleagues.

For example, there were requests for components to be used in the head and neck region, and Brånemark's own particular interest in orthopedics was also an active area of research. Also, by the late 1970s, Kuikka had retired, so there was a pressing need to train and recruit other technicians capable of working with titanium.

With so much learned about titanium – how to work with and handle the metal and mechanical aspects about its design such as surface profile, surface treatment, and tolerances – it seemed enough information was available to make the transition from laboratory to factory. All the lessons had been learned by Kuikka and his small team of technicians over the years. It seemed a relatively straightforward idea to transfer those skills to the more business-oriented atmosphere of a production environment.

The Move to Commercial Production

The same year the Institute was founded, 1978, Brånemark gave the rights to manufacture the titanium components for osseointegration to Bofors, a Swedish company that was mainly known for its weapon business.

Until this point, Brånemark had been in negotiation with a number of Swedish companies. He preferred that the manufacturing license go to a Swedish company, if possible, to facilitate collaboration and communication through geographical proximity. In addition to this, Brånemark felt any manufacturing partner should have a high degree of expertise. Companies with which Brånemark held talks included Astra, a pharmaceutical company, and Aga, one of the world's leading industrial gases groups. At one time Aga appeared to be a particularly promising potential partner. It had begun to diversify from its core business in gas supply and had created or acquired a number of high technology subsidiaries. Negotiations were progressing well, when suddenly Aga announced it had decided not to pursue the project further. Aga's period of rationalization had halted. Indeed, it went into reverse as it divested itself of all its advanced technology following a decision to focus once more on its main or "core" business areas. By contrast, Bofors was at an early phase of a diversification process brought about by the desire to move away from heavy reliance on selling armaments. The Swedish government, partly rocked by a number of arms scandals at that time, felt uncomfortable that a country priding itself on its role in brokering peace around the world should be home to one of the most successful armament companies. At face value, Bofors appeared to have much to offer Brånemark from an engineering perspective. Manufacture of arms requires a high degree of mechanical precision and fine tolerances, just what was needed for the titanium components. Following lengthy discussions, an agreement to create a new enterprise to enter the dental equipment market was made.

In 1981, a company was founded and named Bofors Nobelpharma, with 75 percent ownership by Bofors and 25 percent by the Swedish investment bank, Sveriges Investeringsbank.

In preparation for this company, a project team had been created to bridge the gap between the academic and production worlds. Meetings between the workshop group at the Institute and the new team were intended to provide the information skills transfer needed for production. A production plant at Karlskoga, the site of Bofors' main manufacturing activities, was designated for the production of all the titanium components. During 1982, all the planning and construction for the new manufacturing facility was completed, and production started in 1983.

Problems Along the Way

As is the nature of a new venture, a number of crises and difficulties were experienced in producing components to the standards required for osseointegration. This created a climate of tension and distrust between Brånemark and the management of the new company, which persisted for many years. This experience has also lead Brånemark to campaign strongly for companies working in the health care industries to maintain a strong ethical approach to their businesses. When a company's products end up inside a patient, that company has a strong moral responsibility to maintain the highest standards of quality, precision, and service. The consequences for failure to do so are clear. Apart from effects on an individual patient, which are unconscionable, the long-term implications for a business and the field in which it operates are potentially catastrophic.

The poor history of attempts to introduce dental implant technology prior to Brånemark's work was also a stark reminder of such dangers. Strong adverse perceptions about dental implants were still deeply held by most dental practitioners at the time. Brånemark was justifiably anxious that none of these negative perceptions should be associated with his techniques or the components and equipment needed to apply them in clinical applications. To Brånemark, this meant an uncompromising approach to manufacturing quality and hygiene standards.

During the initial setup and early period of production, Brånemark insisted all components

coming out of the Karlskoga plant be inspected by his own staff to ensure that quality and other important manufacturing criteria were met. At one point the entire plant was halted because of sterilization problems.

Eventually, the production met with Brånemark's approval, though he remained concerned that any business working in the medical field maintain the highest business ethics. Even today, these concerns remain. Brånemark feels strongly that the clinical success of osseointegration is founded on a number of pillars and with clear responsibilities to ensure that the original philosophy of osseointegration is always followed. Brånemark says it is the production company's responsibility to ensure that precision components are reliable and appropriate equipment is available. Otherwise, the entire enterprise and long-term success of implants is threatened. Any product used in a medical context should not be treated in the same way as those that grace a supermarket shelf.

Company Growth

For the fledgling osseointegration company, the period 1982 to 1985 can be classified as turbulent as it experienced changes of ownership and management, coped with a growing workforce, grappled with establishing itself in a number of markets, and dealt with the continued need to finance new developments and marketing activities. The company did not produce its first profits until 1989, as it had had to invest so much in creating what was essentially a new industry.

By the early 1990s, it was still not clear what direction the company would take. By 1991, a total of 400 million Swedish crowns (approximately US $32 million) had been invested in the company. As well as the dental components, the company also had licenses to manufacture the other medical products linked to osseointegration that had come to clinical application following stringent testing. There were essentially three product ranges: dental components and equipment to perform the procedure, the bone-anchored hearing aid, and components for craniofacial rehabilitation.

Nobelpharma came to a crossroads in the mid-1990s. Its business was heavily dental in nature, and it had added other dental technologies to its product portfolio. The bone-anchored hearing aid and the craniofacial work represented small, though profitable, markets for the company. Both showed the power of osseointegration and its potential in other clinical fields. However, the sheer size of the dental market and the huge potential to be tapped led the company to concentrate wholly on this sector.

With dental applications now clearly the core business, the decision was made to split the company. Ownership changed, and the dental part of the company changed its name to Nobel Biocare and merged with an American dental group, Steri-Oss, in 1999. The merger with this company, which had its own dental implant product that competed with the Brånemark system, gave the group around 40 percent of the world market for dental implants.

The bone-anchored hearing aid and the craniofacial work was now marketed by Entific Medical Systems, a new company set up to specialize in this area of osseointegration. The basic principles of the company's business concept have not changed. They are to continue to develop new rehabilitation methods based on the technology and expertise the company already has. Ownership of Entific includes a major shareholding by Nobel Biocare. Other shareholders are the venture capitalist companies Swedestart and Novare Kapital. Clinicians who have seen the dramatic improvement in quality of life for their patients hope the company will get the resources it needs to treat a greater number of patients. Over the past 10 years, approximately 5,000 people have been treated with the osseointegrated retention system for the anchorage of facial prostheses, and more than 6,000 people have been fitted with the bone-anchored hearing aid. Entific has experienced strong growth since the split and by 2001 employed approximately 70 people worldwide, with strong growth in the United States. For this company, gaining official approval for the bone-anchored hearing aid from the US Food and Drug Administration was a major breakthrough.

Current and Potential Markets

The dental applications of osseointegration have experienced strong growth and strong competition. Potentially there is a huge market for dental implants. In the United Kingdom alone, the *Lancet* estimated that in 1990 there were 15 million people who were missing their own teeth in a total population of approximately 56 million.

By the year 2000, a large number of competing implant systems around the world had become established. Most were based in North America, which was the largest market. Many claimed to offer similar results to the Brånemark system. In 1998, the global implant market had reached $450 million, growing at an average annual rate of 10 percent. The largest players at that time were the Brånemark system supplied by Nobel Biocare at 27 percent market share, Steri-Oss at 13 percent, 3i at 13 percent, and ITI at 12 percent.

Penetration of the procedure into the world health care market is patchy because of the huge variations in funding for osseointegration among the particular national health systems. Considering the number of implants per 10,000 people shows the highest penetration in Sweden, with 44 implants per 10,000, followed by Italy and Switzerland.

Such statistics reveal startling facts. While the United States, in 1998, was the largest market based purely on number of implants, the penetration rate was only 16.5 implants per 100,000 people. Japan and the United Kingdom, with their dense populations, also have relatively low penetration rates. Italy has twelve times the market penetration of the United Kingdom and twice the penetration of the United States. Absolute numbers of implants used reveal the three largest markets to be the United States with 420,000 implants, Italy with 210,000, and Germany with 51,000. Looking at the potential for penetration, based on what has already been achieved in Sweden, the total world market could be as high as $1.5 billion.

Local factors have a strong influence on the adoption of any new treatment regime. International variables, the level of government funding, provider training, experience and attitude, and whether or not such treatment is provided by a specialist or generalist must all be considered. In Italy, for example, most osseointegration treatment is provided by a general practitioner. There are also differences in cultural and economic values. Any population receiving such direct services needs the discretionary income to afford them.

Maintaining Standards

As discussed previously, it was originally only the osseointegration system created by Brånemark that was backed up by clear clinical evidence of its efficacy and safety. While Brånemark and others working in osseointegration are pleased that patients have a wider choice of treatments, they are concerned about the uncontrolled and unregulated growth of so-called implantology. One of the keys to the early success of the osseointegration work as it moved into wider application was Brånemark's insistence that individuals and teams embarking upon treating people should be properly trained and deemed competent to carry out the work. Dental practices could not purchase any components and equipment without attending a recognized course on osseointegration and should be supervised in carrying out initial procedures.

This helps set the highest standards in clinical care and provides the optimum conditions for the patient. With percentage success rates in the high 90s for osseointegrated components in both jaws, this insistence has been justified. What puts this success in jeopardy is the increase in practitioners carrying out procedures that do not conform to the same standards or adhere to safe, proven methods.

Professor Patrik Henry, based in Perth, Australia, who carried out some of the early duplicate studies on osseointegration, expresses this concern: "There are always dangers as osseointegration becomes adopted by a broader category within the dental fraternity worldwide, some of whom may lack the training and discipline required to carry out the technique in a predictable way."

Even more critically, he says, "It is important to be aware there exists a small body of practitioners who apply the veneer of osseointegra-

tion but whose motives may more be driven by profit than providing predictable performance. This is a matter of great concern and must not be underestimated. The dental profession and the industry that supplies the tools and equipment should be vigilant about the danger these individuals present."

This is a stark warning, and Henry has also pointed out that the medical product industry has heavy responsibilities to protect the patient, as this can also affect their own long-term survival if products and procedures do not live up to their advertising promises.

"There are ethical issues in business such as truthfulness, fidelity, and beneficence. Products that are not proven to be reliable should not be introduced by industry. Advertising should not be misleading," states Henry. A classic example of this was a temporomandibular joint replacement popular in the United States during the early to mid-1980s. It was found to produce a damaging giant-cell reaction within the temporomandibular joint as a result of breakdown of the Teflon coating. This caused localized tissue destruction and pain. To avoid similar unintended disasters, the implant industry must value research, development, and testing before marketing any products.

In 1999, Henry said, "An important ethical principle is fidelity and commitment both to the patient and health provider. It is important that those businesses supplying products for osseointegration purposes should aim for dependable service and support to clinicians. The basic of business, of any business, is, of course, to make money for its owners and shareholders. Business profitability is important and a measurement of success. Ideally, the patient is treated fairly by the provider and industry when it comes to the overall cost of treatment."

Brånemark has warned about the dangers associated with companies who "concentrate on short-term profit and minute detail differences for the next spring or fall fashion collection according to arbitrary market investigations or anticipations." These concerns point out that those truly committed to osseointegration cannot be complacent about developments done in its name.

Making Osseointegration Accessible

One of Brånemark's preoccupations has been to consider ways of making osseointegration more accessible and affordable for those who could benefit from it. Currently, both the availability and cost of osseointegration treatment have wide variations. Fees vary dramatically between countries, with highest fees appearing to be recorded in Hong Kong, Switzerland, Japan, and the United Kingdom. The average fee for a fixed bridge can range from a low of approximately US $5,000 to more than US $20,000 in Hong Kong. Clearly, osseointegration services are expensive, which limits their application. One of Brånemark's goals in the coming years was to broaden the categories of patients who have access to the treatment and to overcome the local, financial, and other difficulties that prevent this from being achieved. As a result, in May 1999, Brånemark and his colleagues introduced Novum, a "same-day teeth" concept designed to shorten the time and reduce the cost of providing fixed dental prostheses.

Novum, which is described in more detail in Chapter 4, demands a high level of precision and is a very unforgiving procedure in the respect that adherence to the method and correct use of appropriate equipment is paramount. That said, both the knowledge and equipment designs exist, and the only obstacle appears to be the commercial will to manufacture and deliver the Novum components and associated instrumentation as specified. So far the industrial response to this breakthrough has been disappointing because the dental sector has not appeared to realize the significance and potential of this approach to treat broad categories of patients worldwide.

Clinical Applications of Osseointegration

Part II

4 Transformations in Dentistry

"That action is best, which procures the greatest happiness for the greatest numbers."

Francis Hutcheson, 1694-1746

As stated in Part I, dental applications of osseointegration were initially considered only for those patients who could not be treated by any other means. However, after demonstrating that osseointegration was successful, it became apparent that it could be applied to a large range of dental procedures from a single-tooth replacement to patients who are completely edentulous.

There is no doubt that osseointegration has changed the nature of clinical restorative dentistry. In the 1990s, there was an increasing emphasis on esthetics and prosthetics. This has resulted in continuing refinements and redefinitions in osseointegration.

The scope of osseointegration in dentistry should not be forgotten. It allows the treatment of all ages and categories of patients, it can replace a single tooth or all, correct small or large defects, and be used for simple or complicated procedures. Osseointegration has proved itself a very successful technology with few drawbacks – the biological price is a small loss of bone.

Cost of Osseointegration

Despite the proven success of osseointegration in dental applications, its demonstrated long-term benefits, and its good functional and esthetic results, osseointegration remains a technique applied to less than 1 percent of dental patients. It is true that dental companies offering implants have experienced strong growth and strong competition. Potentially there is a huge market for dental implants, yet osseointegration remains the preserve of the few. It can only be used when either the health care system or the patient can absorb the relatively high cost of treatment. In the United Kingdom, for example, many patients are faced with considerable bills for a visit to the dentist as it lies outside the coverage of the essentially free medical health system. Those who visit the increasingly rare National Health Service- (NHS) funded dentists must bear 80 percent of the costs. For the more unusual treatments, and even when several crowns are required, NHS permission must be granted before the work can be carried out. Implants often lie outside that funding anyway, so individuals must have the resources to pay for the entire procedure themselves.

Superior Performance

Any attempt to make comparisons between osseointegration and conventional dentistry has to be mindful of the relatively low numbers of patients treated with osseointegration globally. Considering a single-tooth bonded bridge, the 4-year longevity rate is 75 percent, of which the maxillary failure rate ranges from 22 to 27 percent and the mandibular rate from 20 to 56 percent. For a fixed bridge, the average longevity is 12 to 15 years. Of those failures that do occur, around 70 percent are mechanical in origin. Removable partial dentures have a poor record with 50 percent never worn by patients. So this is not a good therapeutic result.

Patrik Henry has pointed out that the superior performance of osseointegration in dental applications, compared to other treatment systems, has been confirmed in a number of multicenter studies. When osseointegration is compared to traditional prosthodontics, its long-term success rates reveal its superiority to conventional alternatives. For the single tooth, the totally or partially edentulous jaw, maxillofacial applications, and for the emerging orthodontic applications, osseointegration is clearly superior. That said, there are a number of hurdles that continue to hamper the growth of osseointegration to replace traditional procedures. Cost, availability, and suitably trained practitioners are the three major factors.

Despite these problems, the potential of osseointegration in other areas of dentistry continues to be explored. Henry has commented that he and his colleagues are now extrapolating the bone-anchorage possibilities in the orthodontic fields into various other applications. One example is to use implants in the basal bone to reposition jaws as an alternative to orthognathic surgery. Implants are placed in the zygomatic arches, and, using a facial appliance, the maxilla is gradually pulled downward and forward. This procedure takes 6 months moving the maxilla at a rate of 1 mm per month with no surgical intervention. This is an exciting development at the leading edge of dental technology.

Broader Dental Applications

As dental applications involving osseointegration have become more routine, new ways of providing treatment have become appropriate. Increasingly, cases that were once considered too severe or in need of a complicated range of procedures can now benefit from recent developments in osseointegration. In the case of the edentulous, severely resorbed maxilla, the development of a long fixture, the zygomaticus fixture, allows anchorage in the zygoma. This bone can be reached by going through the sinus without complications. Originally, this technique was developed to overcome difficulties in patients with major craniofacial and oral defects where bone was lacking (Figs 4-1a and 4-1b). Cases treated with this fixture have had successful outcomes with few observed problems, similar to patients treated for the more complicated maxillofacial problems.

For all types of treatment, osseointegration relies on precision surgery, good prosthetics, and reliable components. As the competence and awareness of the procedures have grown, the nature and environment in which osseointegration is practiced have changed.

Originally, strong teams were required to ensure that the strict rules were applied and maintained. While the importance of the team approach has always been emphasized by Per-Ingvar Brånemark, in recent years individual dentists have been trained and are able to suc-

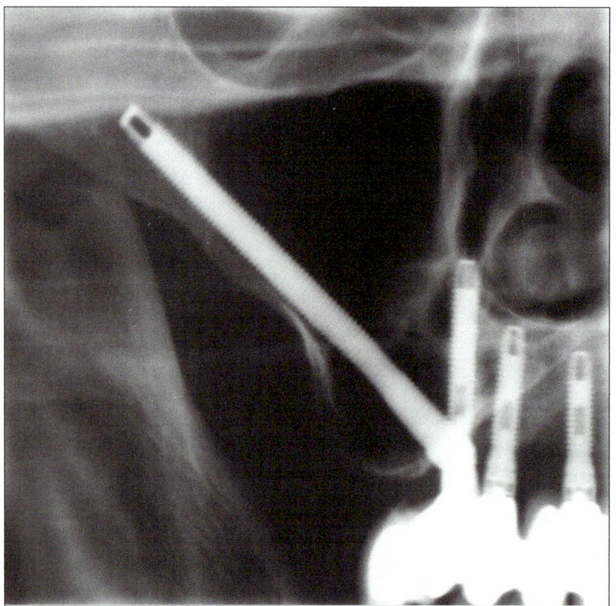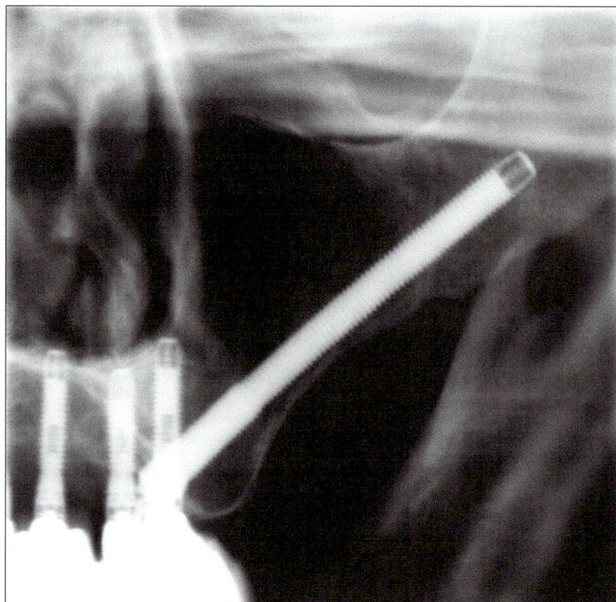

Figs 4-1a and **4-1b** One example of the ability to adapt osseointegration to suit patient needs. The zygomaticus fixture can provide support for those patients with little bone, avoiding the need for additional bone grafting in some cases, even for a severely resorbed maxilla.

cessfully apply osseointegration for single teeth on their own. This does not negate the importance of the team approach; it simply provides an alternative that will be monitored over the long term. This is one way of bringing down the costs of treatment for the individual, which is a necessary step if osseointegration is to reach the greater community.

Osseointegration in dentistry will, over the next few years, undergo changes in diagnosis and treatment. It is predicted that there will be a breakthrough in the application of osseointegration to the public at large.

"Today the state of the art in dentistry is osseointegration. If we are to offer optimized management to our patients that will mean osseointegration. How the health delivery system deals with the provision of osseointegration to a wider audience than before is the main issue for debate," Henry said at a conference in 1999.

By the year 2000, 1.2 million patients had been treated using the Brånemark system. One of the factors behind Brånemark's success as a researcher is that he continually questions the way things are done, even in respect to his own work. On May 2, 1999, Brånemark announced yet another development in the history of dental osseointegration: the concept of providing a new set of teeth for the mandible in a single day. This is Novum.

Novum: New Teeth in a Day

Brånemark has always been convinced that the provision of dental rehabilitation should be as simple and as affordable as possible. He feels that too often people are guided, or blinded, by the philosophy that extensive treatment — whether surgical or prosthetic — is for a small, affluent percentage of the global population. Many millions of edentulous individuals suffer just as much from their handicap, but sadly lack both the means and accessibility to implant treatment.

Novum is a step toward broader access for those who are completely edentulous in either or both maxilla and mandible. In Sweden the cost of providing a new set of fixed teeth using the Novum concept is 17,000 Swedish crowns (around £1,200 or US $2,000), which includes all the surgical procedures and materials. This is quite a reasonable cost when compared to other prosthetic treatments of similar quality. In addition, the hope is that this cost can be reduced further through a contribution from the Swedish national health insurance system.

The Novum development is based on precision surgery with a range of standard prefabricated guides and components suitable for use with the majority of patients (Figs 4-2 to 4-5). Though the surgery is fairly demanding, the prosthetic requirements are straightforward and simple. No individual impressions are needed as all the components fit together in the same way for each patient, and no temporary components need to be used. The Novum concept is based on rigidly connecting and then loading the implants at the time of insertion. This is believed to produce biological benefits in terms of bone remodeling and for the final loading situation.

For a number of years, Brånemark and Richard Skalak had discussed the idea of simplified treatment. The biomechanical requirements of an immediate loading concept in the mandible were assessed as long ago as 1980, and prototype designs were evaluated in 1995. The mandible is considered to have less complicated demands than the maxilla, in terms of anatomy and biological prerequisites. These evaluations and subsequent modifications took about a year, by which time the group felt that preliminary clinical evaluation was safe to begin.

In February 1996, the first set of patients was treated using the same-day concept. Through September of that year, a total of 150 patients were treated. They were followed over a 3-year period, and they participated in a clinical study whose results were complete by the end of 2000. Preliminary results showed that bone integration had taken place in 98 percent of cases, with excellent bridge stability in 99 percent of patients. In a 3-year study carried out at the Brånemark Osseointegration Center in Gothenburg, of 270 fixtures inserted in 90 patients, only 3 such components were lost. Also, of the patients interviewed so far, 95 percent had not reported any problems with their new teeth and were able to begin eating by the first evening following treatment.

Initially, the treatment was split into different sections and took place over a period of a week.

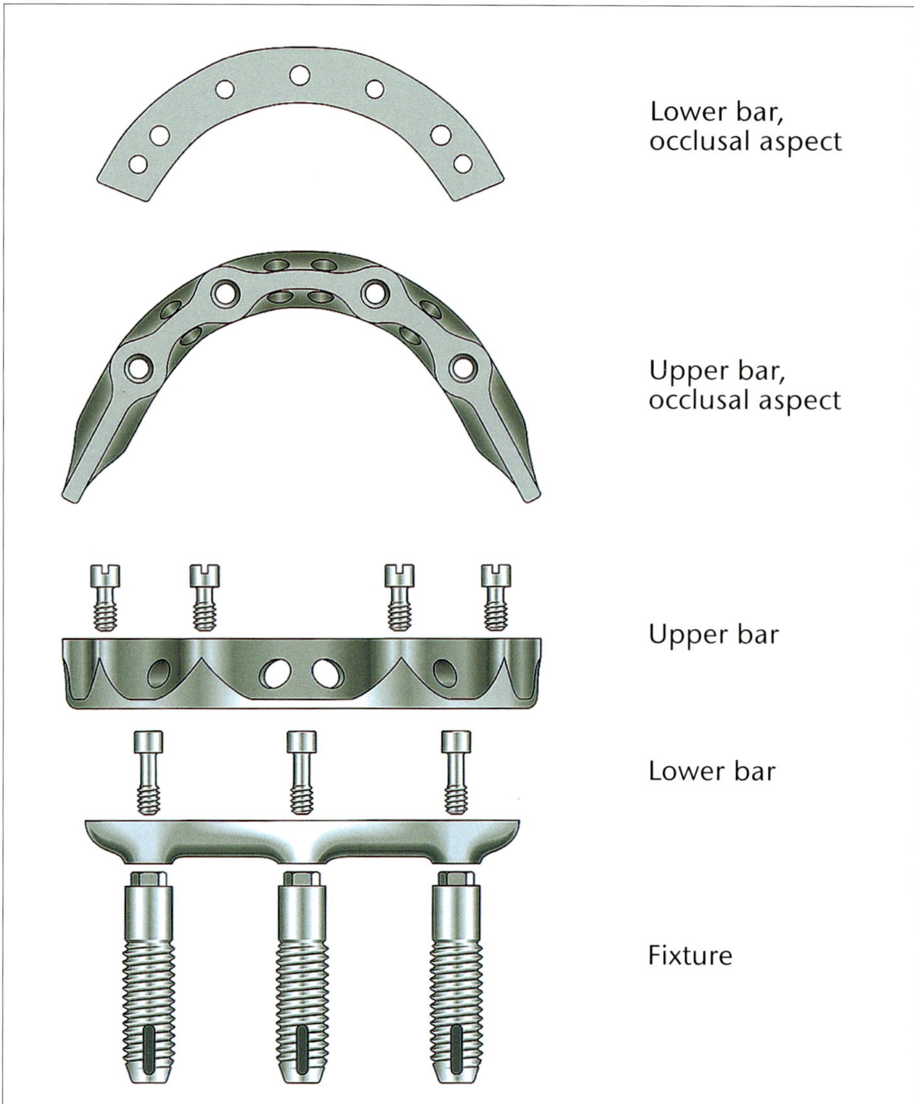

Fig 4-2 Prefabricated precision components allow the Novum system to be adapted to each patient for a reasonable cost. The time taken to provide a dental prosthesis is shortened to a single day.

No unexpected problems arose, and gradually, the elements of the procedure were performed over shorter timeframes, eventually meeting the single-day requirement.

The Novum treatment is carried out as follows. The patient comes to the clinic in the morning and radiographs are taken frontally, laterally, and axially to provide preoperative information about the seating of the titanium fixtures. Additional seating details use two fixed points – one at the forehead and one on the cheek to provide the "bite height."

The three titanium fixtures are inserted with the aid of a surgical template placed over the mandible. Then the mucous membrane is closed, and a base plate is placed over the tita-nium screws. This ensures that there is no contralateral movement that would hinder osseointegration between the bone and the fixtures. The prefabricated bridge construction is fixed above and to the base plate. The surgical procedure itself takes about 1.5 hours. Impressions and other remedial procedures are not required as the prefabricated design suits around 95 percent of patients.

Though the surgical procedure takes slightly longer than the procedures with standard components, there are other savings. It has been estimated that overall, the one-stage procedure means 70 percent less "chair time" for the patient and an 80 percent lower surgical fee. Overall, this all adds up to a 50 percent savings compared to

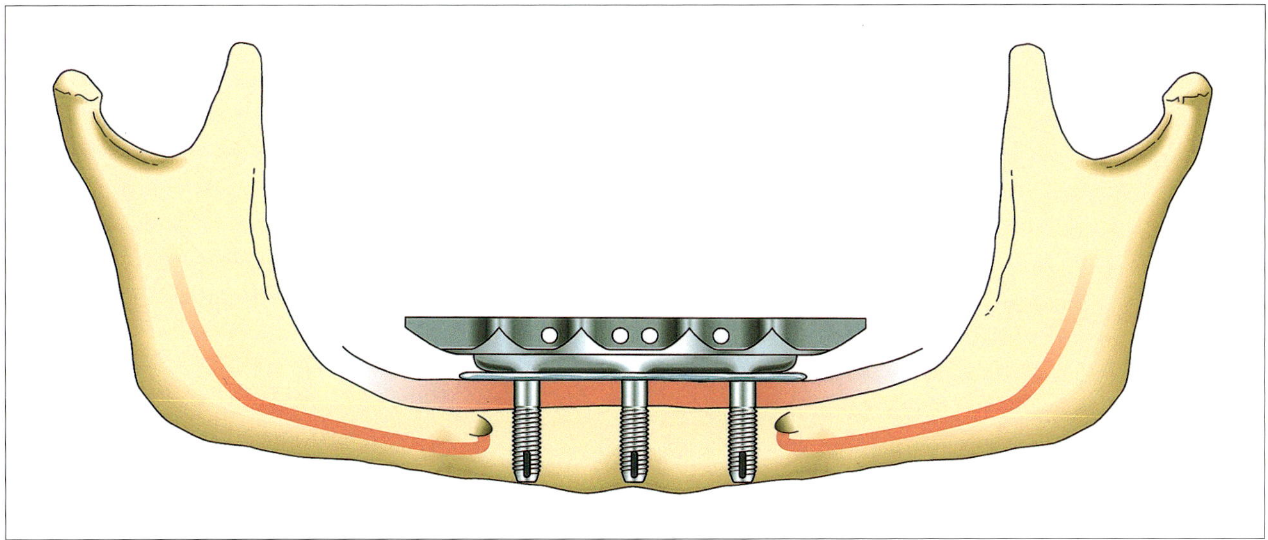

Fig 4-3 The sub- and superstructures are designed to fit together accurately.

existing osseointegration procedures. Though the surgical procedure is more demanding, the prosthetic procedure is far simpler.

In July 2000, the first patients were treated in the maxilla using the Novum concept, and the expectations are that the same high success rate – well in excess of 90 percent – will be achieved for this procedure. Brånemark notes the further potential for this technology, "Modification of the mandibular procedure as well as further adaptation and application for various other types of edentulism might be possible."

The hope is that Novum will become more generally available. Multicenter studies are already underway, as is an educational program to inform other clinicians about the potential of the technique.

The initial response from other practitioners in Sweden, and increasingly at centers around the world, has been extremely positive. Some regard it as marking a new and exciting era in the field of osseointegration. Since the turn of the millennium, Brånemark and his team have been traveling around the world, teaching and demonstrating the technique at specialist centers worldwide. Novum has the potential to rekindle excitement in the implant dentistry world, as well as offer treatment to a broader spectrum of individuals. There remains the question, though, of whether commercial entities have the commitment, expertise, and vision to realize the tremendous potential of this technique.

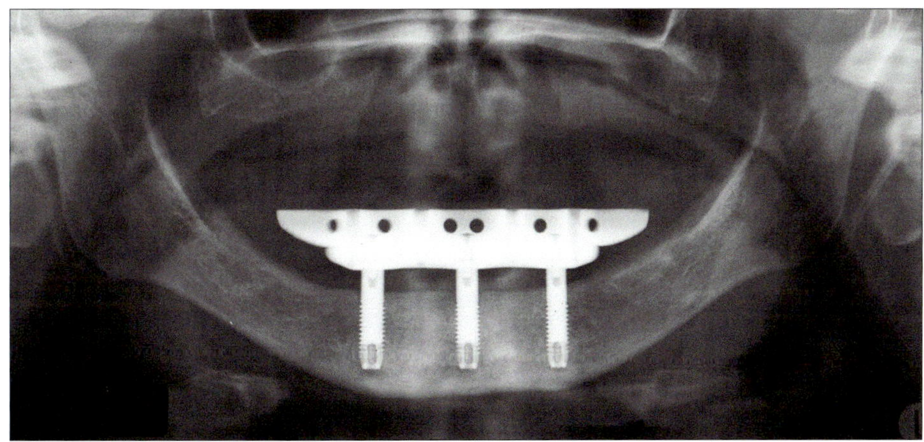

Fig 4-4 A typical panoramic radiograph showing the topographical position of the anchoring fixtures in relation to the anatomy of the mandible.

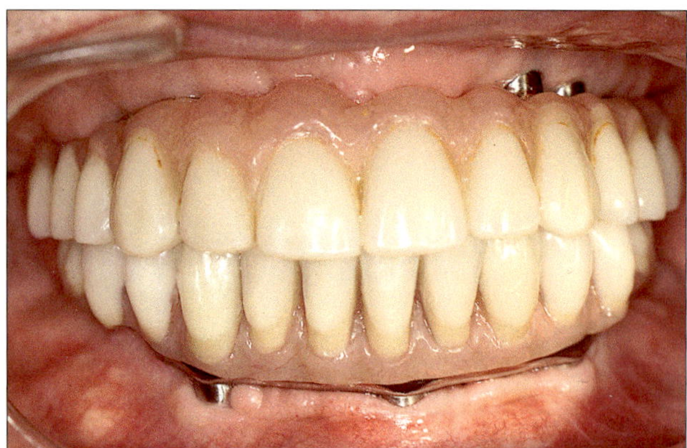

Fig 4-5 This patient has been treated using the Novum single-day concept with both practical and esthetically pleasing results.

Brånemark fears the lessons so painstakingly learned during the development and subsequent manufacture of the original titanium components and osseointegration equipment have not been taken to corporate heart. During the development of the Novum technique, Brånemark worked with Nobel Biocare so this company would have all the information to develop the production resources for the commercialization of the same-day teeth concept.

Bearing in mind that clinical trials began in 1996 and yielded successful results around the world, the potential market for this concept is clearly evident. It was with growing frustration that Brånemark realized Nobel Biocare had been unable to deliver, or was not interested in delivering, suitable equipment to carry out the technique. In June 2000, this prompted Brånemark to comment, "The basic problems are precision and priorities concerning components and instruments. For reasons beyond our control and understanding, the responsible commercial company has not managed to deliver adequate and reliable equipment within reasonable time." Further Brånemark believes he has no choice but to restrict his application of the Novum treatment modality to the edentulous mandible for the time being because of the "severely reluctant attitude from the commercial company." His hope was that the necessary hardware for this treatment would become available by the year 2001, though the prospects for this were increasingly bleak, and he is still waiting.

However, the difference in philosophy and difficulties in communication between Brånemark and commercial forces continue to be the main sticking point in the further development of osseointegration in the dental context. Once again, Brånemark and his colleagues find themselves in a deeply frustrating situation where a promising treatment regime that could be used to provide an affordable solution to edentulism is delayed by the procrastination of a business that fails to see the commercial benefits of investing in new technology.

Facing the World

"Two men look out through the same bars; one sees the mud, and one the stars."
Thomas Henry Huxley, 1825-1895

Most humans are concerned about their appearance. Though differences in culture and social custom may produce different perceptions about the nature of beauty and fashion, humans desire to be regarded as having socially acceptable features. Conforming to norms helps with our social development and interaction, as well as our personal confidence.

To some degree, we all fret about the imperfections of our own bodies and the ravages imposed upon it by passing time. We may note, with some guilty satisfaction, the encroaching wrinkles on some famous beauty whose attributes we have always coveted. Such is the nature of the human soul.

Increasingly, those with the financial resources are turning to plastic surgery as a way of delaying the effects of age or improving various aspects of their bodies. Increasingly, individuals are not afraid to seek cosmetic treatment to improve their appearance. Many of the social taboos surrounding such treatment have disappeared. People desire to maintain or improve their looks because of the perfect images of models that bombard their senses in the media. Though plastic surgery is often regarded as a tool used for essentially vain purposes, another use is far more serious and laudable — to rehabilitate those who have suffered a variety of disfiguring and disabling problems. The fact that plastic surgery is becoming more widely available reveals that the techniques are becoming more predictable and reliable for straightforward cases and that experience has been gained for more complex and challenging cases.

Today the term plastic surgery encompasses a wide range of treatments and surgical options. It includes, for example, conventional and osseointegrated prosthetics to autologous reconstruction, transplants, and the latest technology in the form of tissue engineering.

Modern plastic surgery owes the impetus for its development to the damage inflicted upon those fighting in World War II. Surgeons had the task of trying to rehabilitate patients with horrendous facial burns, blast victims, and those with lost limbs.

The Challenge of Facial Damage

In many ways, each case is unique when it comes to facial problems. Patients range, for example, from the child born without ears to the middle-aged woman whose face was damaged in a car crash. There is the case of the young woman whose life and face were destroyed by a gunshot from a crazed stranger, the patient whose face was distorted by cancer, or the person whose features were removed in an industrial accident. Their stories and circumstances are all heartrending. As well as changed features, these events leave individuals with an altered outlook on living in society, where so many judgments depend on appearance.

In many ways, facial reconstruction remains a considerable challenge to the plastic surgeon. The medical team is faced with a number of issues in the treatment of the patients, particularly those who have suffered trauma or cancer that has resulted in the destruction of facial features. Those living with a changed appearance not only have to overcome their own feelings of loss and horror but also have to deal with the distaste and embarrassment that they engender in others. While any caring, compassionate society should be sensitive to people in such situations, it is sadly true that those who do not conform to perceived normal appearance are often shunned or ostracized. Often such patients withdraw completely from interaction with the outside world.

For cancer or trauma patients, surgeons' responsibilities need to go beyond the initial life-saving procedures to support the patient by restoring quality of life through rehabilitation. The point at which rehabilitation starts is related to the patient's own physical and mental condition and the approach taken by the surgeon. There are a number of philosophical and practical considerations to be taken into account. The treatment team has to tread a very delicate professional line. The psychological state of the patient has to be carefully assessed. Cancer sufferers, in particular, are in a very vulnerable psychological state. It is important that such patients are fully informed about the nature of their condition and accept their situation and the prognosis. The patient needs to understand that it is not possible to completely restore features or function to their pre-cancer condition either through implant treatment or any other rehabilitation regime.

In Gothenburg, all the members of the rehabilitation team work closely together, when possible. In some instances, where a cancer patient is to have resection at the same hospital, the rehabilitation team may have the opportunity to see the patient before surgery takes place. Communication between the surgical and the rehabilitation team can help with the planning of the surgery to take into account the optimal conditions for rehabilitation. For example, in the case of a shallow orbital defect, the rehabilitation team may suggest that the defect be deepened slightly to better accommodate the prosthetic framework and the associated silicone design. The rehabilitation team can provide guidance about not only the size and depth of the defect but its shape and contour. The team might also request, when possible, that eyebrows be preserved to help mask the presence of the prosthesis.

The Gothenburg rehabilitation team has also found that early contact with a patient before radical surgery has a number of benefits. It is positive to patients from a psychological perspective in that it can give them a sense of hope. It can mark the fact that rehabilitation is already being considered at a time when patients are feeling vulnerable and fearful for the future. The chance for the rehabilitation team to see a patient before radical procedures also allows them to create a prosthesis that will mirror more closely the individual's original features.

Prosthetic Solutions

Where possible, plastic surgeons' first choice of treatment is to repair damage using tissue grafts from the patient. After all, the best solution would be to replace malformed, damaged, or lost tissue in a cosmetically attractive way. However, there are a considerable number of occasions where insufficient bone and tissue are available to provide an acceptable prosthetic and functional result.

In some cases, the nature and complication of the plastic surgery, which may involve a number of surgical procedures spread over months and even years, cannot be tolerated emotionally by a patient. In such situations, prosthetics can provide an acceptable replacement of lost facial features. Modern plastics and the advance of prosthetic design technology have yielded life-like replicas of human features, but attaching these prostheses had been a major problem until the advent of osseointegration.

The prosthesis needs to be held firmly in place to provide the wearer with security and confidence, but it has to be removable for cleaning and repair. Solutions to attaching prostheses include cosmetic glue, double-sided tape, and magnets. In the eye and nose regions, glasses can be used to hold prostheses. The problem with these methods is the constant worry to the patient that the prosthesis may come loose. Patients have recorded a number of embarrassing and distressing incidents. One patient, on her first social outing in a restaurant with friends and family, had to retrieve her prosthetic nose from a bowl of tomato soup. The heat of the soup had melted the cosmetic glue that held the device. In that single moment, all the confidence and courage that had brought her to that point was destroyed.

Osseointegration offers a straightforward and effective answer to retention of craniofacial

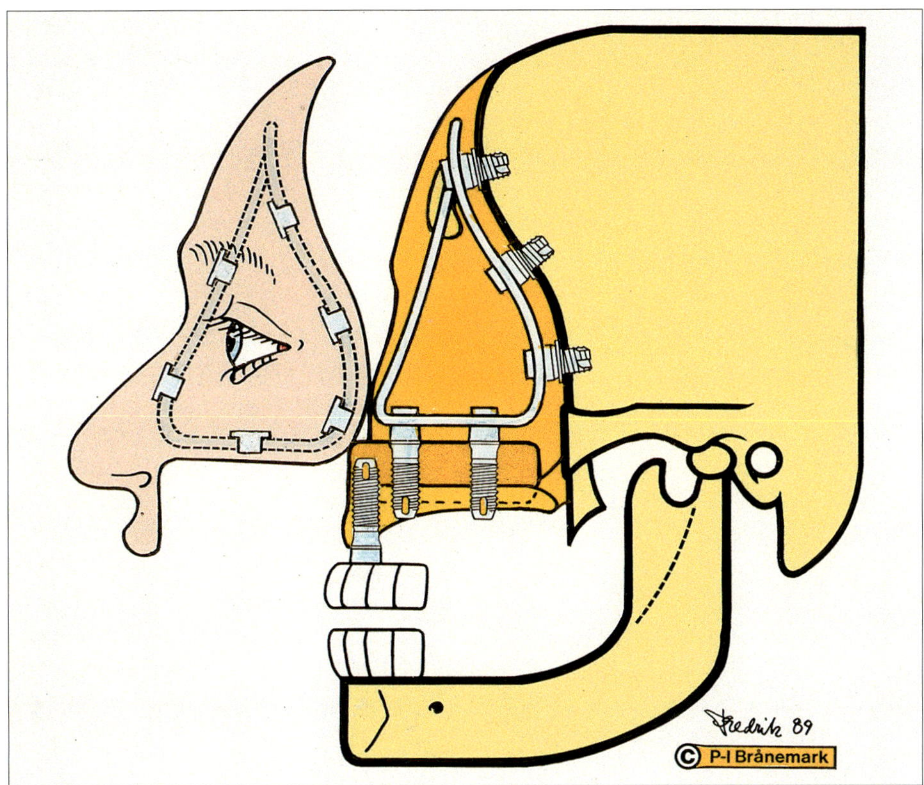

Fig 5-1 The proposition for a functional facial prosthesis in the mid-face region. Bone-anchored fixtures provide the platform for a three-part prosthesis to provide dentition in the maxilla, to create an artificial palate, and to provide anchorage for a facial mask.

prostheses. The nature of the technology means it can handle both simple and complex designs. Equally important, the technique is designed so it does not preclude the use of plastic surgery or other rehabilitation methods, should results of these alternatives offer a better solution for patients (Fig 5-1).

Early Applications of Osseointegration

The first application of osseointegration for prosthetic retention was a relatively straightforward procedure to support an artificial pinna, or outer ear. In 1982, Sven Ljungkvist had cancer in the outer ear, which was surgically removed. Surgeon Anders Tjellström, who worked in the ear, nose, and throat (ENT) department at Sahlgren's University Hospital in Gothenburg, carried out the procedure with Brånemark.

The procedure was based on the two-step system developed for dental applications of osseointegration. This meant an interval of 3 to 4 months between the insertion of the fixtures and the addition of the skin-penetrating abutments. Normally, for an ear replacement, two or three titanium fixtures are placed in the mastoid. The positioning of the fixtures in relation to the external ear canal is key to providing the best cosmetic result. At the second stage, a few months later, the sites of components are identified, and the skin and tissue covering these fixtures carefully opened. This allows skin-penetrating abutments or cylinders to be attached using titanium screws and, to prevent inflammatory processes at the site of the abutment, the skin is trimmed and connected to the periosteum, according to a method suggested by Professor Olle Hallén. Over these fixtures, a small retention bar is connected and onto this construction, the prosthetic ear can be fixed.

In the same way, osseointegration can provide anchorage points for other facial features. For an eye or nose prosthesis, a minimum of two fixtures inserted into appropriate bone close to the defect can provide support for a life-like prosthesis.

Creating Prostheses

There are a number of stages in the creation of a prosthesis: taking an impression of the defect, making a bar construction, providing an acrylic base plate for the bar, ensuring correct positioning, making a wax model, producing a mold, and adding the final cosmetic touches. The use and fabrication of prostheses goes back many hundreds of years. Ivory and hammered copper are some of the materials from which such devices have been made. There is even the story of a woman in Berlin who, for 40 years, "baked" a new prosthetic nose every day. Today, the majority of prostheses are made of silicones, sometimes combined with metals or other plastics. Silicones are easy to work with and match to individual skin tone. They are not as durable as human skin, so periodic replacement is necessary. Artificial materials deteriorate because they are subject to wear and discoloration from environmental contamination.

Along with the development of the osseointegration technique, adaptations of conventional prosthetic design to suit the new method of attachment were required. Kerstin Bergström, now an associate professor at Gothenburg, was the first maxillofacial prosthetic technician to work in the ENT department of Sahlgren's University Hospital. She joined the department as a dental technician but found "doing only teeth was boring." Luckily, she got the opportunity to get involved with the new osseointegration program. She played a key role in creating this new approach to prosthesis design. Bergström's work in developing acceptable prosthetic designs has been spread throughout the world, thanks to comprehensive training programs in Gothenburg and at other major rehabilitation centers. Even today, all the prosthetic design work is based on the techniques she pioneered, and she continues to play an active role in their development and the training of other professionals. She says it is a tremendous privilege to work with craniofacial patients. The courage, humor, and strength demonstrated by people in the face of such awful disabilities is uplifting and continues to inspire Bergström in her daily work.

In contrast to traditional prosthesis creation, in Bergström's approach, the starting point is a wax model of the feature to be created, which forms the mold for the final silicone prosthesis. Several fittings are needed to ensure that the prosthesis will have a suitable likeness and can match the existing skin texture and tone.

Benefits of Osseointegration

One of the important benefits of an osseointegrated prosthesis is that the maxillofacial technician or anaplastologist has a range of sophisticated retention options, including a bar and clips, bar and magnet, individual magnets, ball attachments, or a combination. The choice of retention mechanism is dependent on the size of the defect, position, orientation, and number of implants. Then there is the consideration of how the fixtures will be loaded to avoid unnecessary stress and movement of facial tissue in relation to the prosthesis.

The same basic principle can be applied to both simple and complex defects. For example, cases that involve the mid-face region present the greatest challenge to the rehabilitation team. Damage to this part of the face often means the ability to talk and eat is impaired, aside from the facial disfigurement. Patients who have experienced extensive loss of palatal, oral, and nasal structures often feel depressed and frustrated by their inability to produce intelligible speech. More devastating is the way they are often regarded by others.

Extensive loss of tissue and bone in the face may mean a combination of treatments is required, including plastic surgery and bone and skin grafts. Complex cases still require the insertion of suitable titanium fixtures at appropriate points in healthy bone, which can provide the anchorage point for the external prosthetic device. Often a patient requires both intraoral and extraoral rehabilitation. There have been a number of successful cases in which patients have been given back their lives.

One long-standing patient was Nils Björkdahl, who had to have radical surgery because of facial cancer. This left him without his left eye, nose, upper lip, upper set of teeth, as well as the bone and soft tissue that covered much of the left side of his face. Björkdahl's rehabilitation program included bone grafting, the creation of an upper lip, and osseointegration that provided him with a functional set of teeth and a method of securing his three-part facial prosthesis (Figs 5-2a to 5-2e). Because of Brånemark's early studies relating to the interaction of bone and marrow tissues, it was routine to use autologous marrow tissues at the anchorage sites to help promote healing, particularly if the tissue had been irradiated.

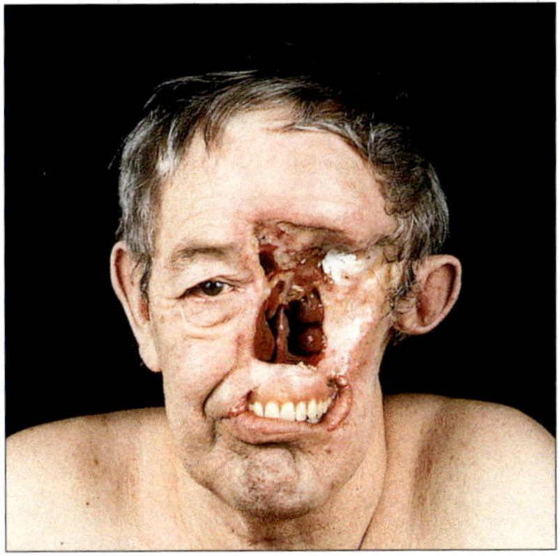

Fig 5-2a Nils Björkdahl's treatment was carried out in a number of stages. Plastic surgery provided him with an upper lip to help support a facial prosthesis.

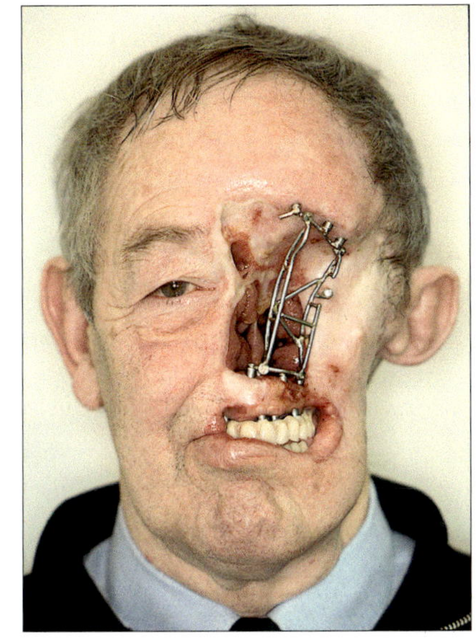

Fig 5-2b An intraoral dental prosthesis was created and a framework for the facial prosthesis was connected to implanted fixtures.

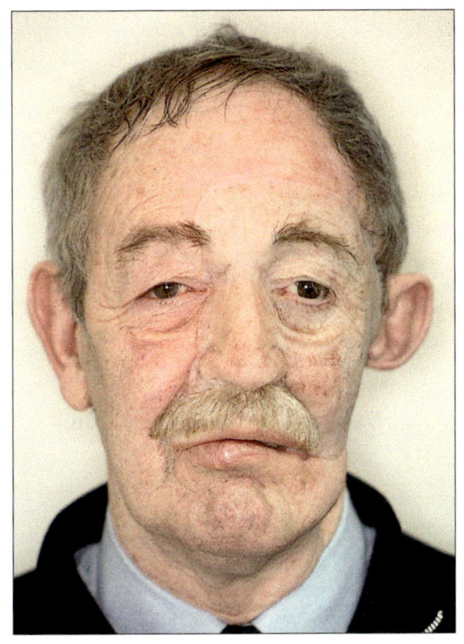

Fig 5-2c With the three-part prosthesis in place, Björkdahl was able to enjoy a good quality of life for many years.

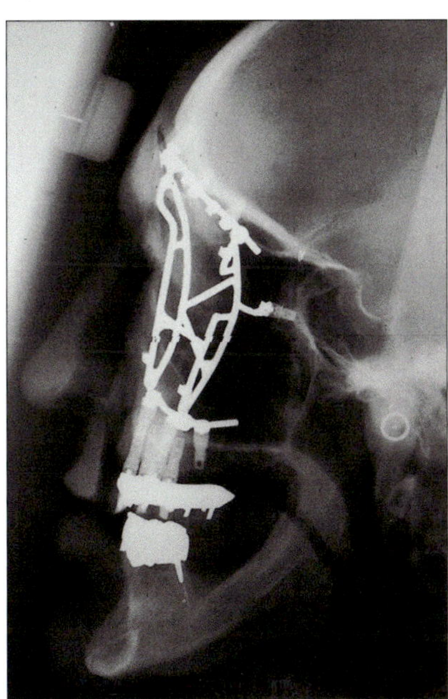

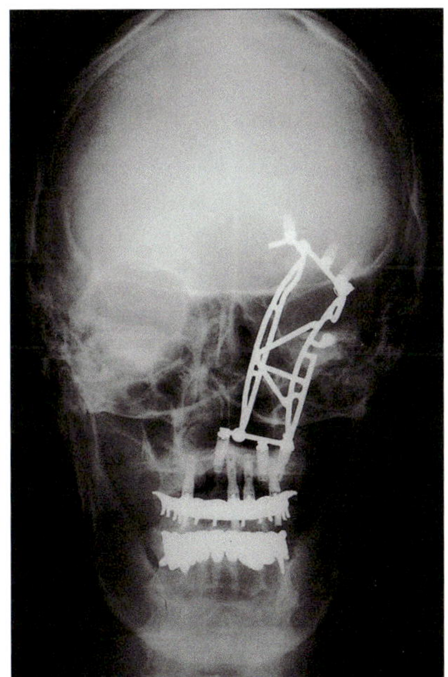

Figs 5-2d and **5-2e** Radiographs showing how Björkdahl's fixtures are placed within his residual facial bone structure.

Once the rehabilitation was completed, Björkdahl reported that his life had been transformed. He was once again able to enjoy an active social life and enjoyed an improved quality of life for a number of years. Over the years, Björkdahl benefited from the improved skills of the anaplastologist. He used to travel to the hospital in a special taxi. On one of his last trips to the clinic when a new prosthesis was made, the taxi driver recalled driving Björkdahl on a previous occasion and noted, "I remember driving you before, but at that time you had a facial mask." Nils was so thrilled by this comment, which revealed he looked normal and was in effect getting a real face back, that he told everyone.

For cancer patients, the need to irradiate bone as part of the treatment regime can have an adverse effect on bone quality. This provides a less favorable prognosis for the survival of titanium fixtures in bone. The highest implant losses have been seen in the supraorbital rim, followed by the lateral orbital rim, mandible, maxilla, and mastoid. Originally, the fact that a patient had been irradiated was a contraindication for osseointegration treatment. That is no longer the case, as patients can have supplementary treatment to improve bone quality. Hyperbaric oxygen treatment, developed by Gösta Granström, prior to osseointegration, improves implant survival rates versus those of non-irradiated patients. Giving patients enriched oxygen treatment is achieved by placing them in a diving chamber, normally used for treating divers suffering from "the bends." Patients are given 20 90-minute sessions in the diving chamber at 2.5 times atmospheric pressure, subsequently followed by first-stage implant surgery and further immediate postoperative hyperbaric oxygen treatment with the equivalent of 10 oxygen dives. The use of autologous marrow tissue again supports healing.

Teams working with complex cases have realized that treatment can have adverse consequences. The treatment plan for difficult cases has to take into account many aspects such as long-term maintenance and monitoring and also include therapeutic reserves that can have unforeseen setbacks.

The general improvement in the treatment and diagnosis of all types of cancer through better diagnostic imaging, therapies, and surgical approaches has benefited cancer patients through higher survival rates and longer lifetimes. In the case of maxillofacial cancer sufferers, this puts pressure on the treatment team to provide ways of improving the quality of life for a group of patients whose prognosis for long-term survival has improved dramatically.

This is amply illustrated by the case of an Australian patient whose appearance was severely damaged by cancer of the mid-face. Radical, life-saving surgery was successful but left him without the ability to communicate, eat properly, or go out in public. He underwent rehabilitation using osseointegration, and the treatment team created a functioning system that transformed this patient's existence. Though this patient has since died because of a recurrence of the disease, the rehabilitation gave him more than a decade with a good quality of life (Figs 5-3a to 5-3j).

Treating such patients does demand huge resources and is regarded as a life-long commitment. Throughout the world, professional teams providing maxillofacial rehabilitation using osseointegration develop a close relationship with individual patients, a relationship that is not generally found in other areas of medicine. Such association with individuals can be uplifting and beneficial to both the treatment team and the patient.

Other Applications for Osseointegration

The use of osseointegrated prostheses is not just for cancer or trauma patients, although these form the majority of cases. There are a number of congenital conditions, such as atresia affecting the ear, that are often appropriate for osseointegration procedures. Atresia is a condition that affects around 1 in 10,000 people. It is sometimes associated with Treacher Collins syndrome sufferers who have hearing loss.

The options for children range from plastic surgery to reconstruct the pinna to an artificial ear attached using osseointegration. A plastic surgery approach pioneered by American surgeon Burt Brent has made dramatic progress in providing an esthetically acceptable outer ear. Still there are occasions when a patient may

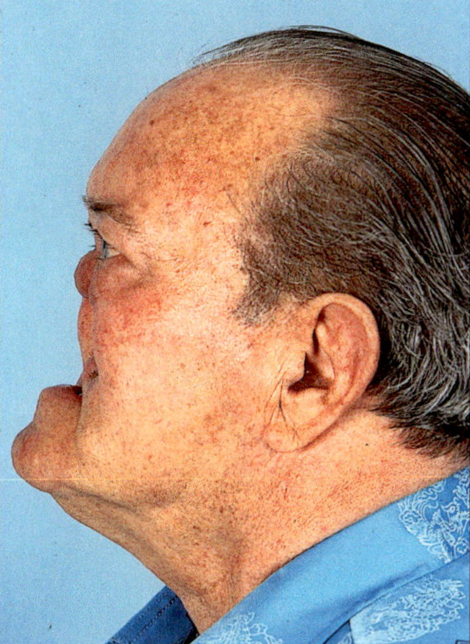

Fig 5-3a Cancer of the mid-face followed by radical surgery that included a maxillectomy left this patient with a considerable facial defect that could not be corrected by plastic surgery.

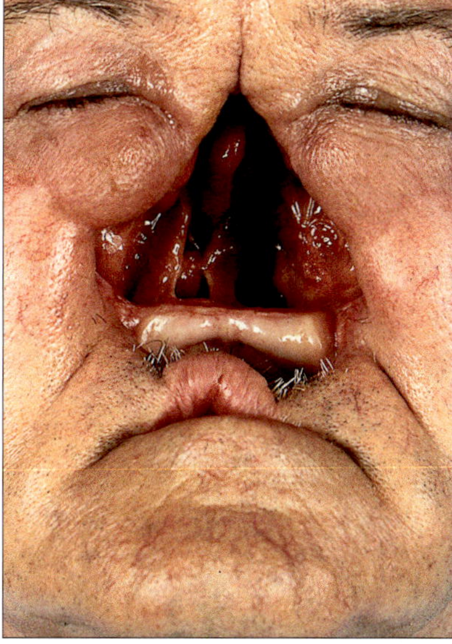

Fig 5-3b The mid-face defect represented a considerable challenge to the rehabilitation team. The first procedure was carried out in April 1994 to provide fixtures for a facial prosthesis and obturator.

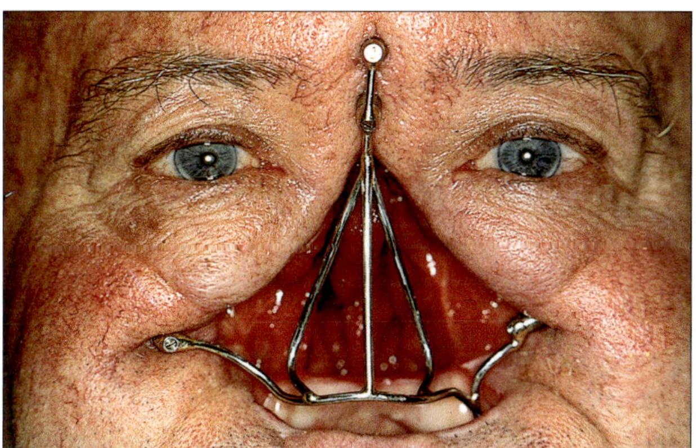

Fig 5-3c Fixtures were inserted into the residual bone and a framework attached.

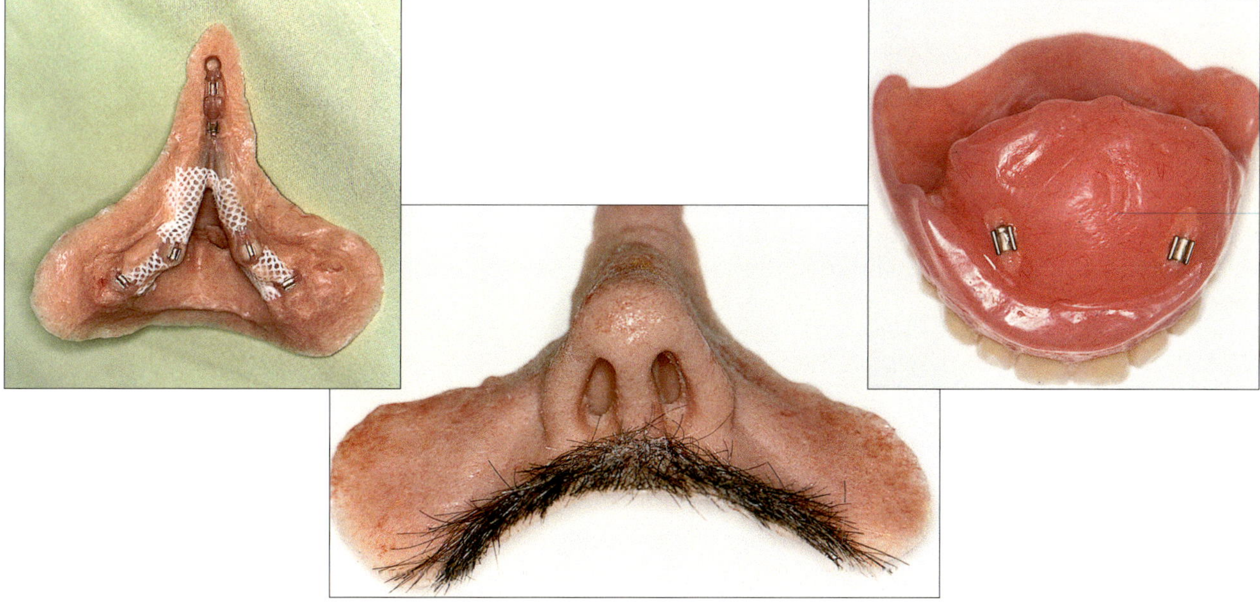

Figs 5-3d to **5-3f** This framework provided anchorage points for dentition, including an artificial palate, and for the facial prosthesis.

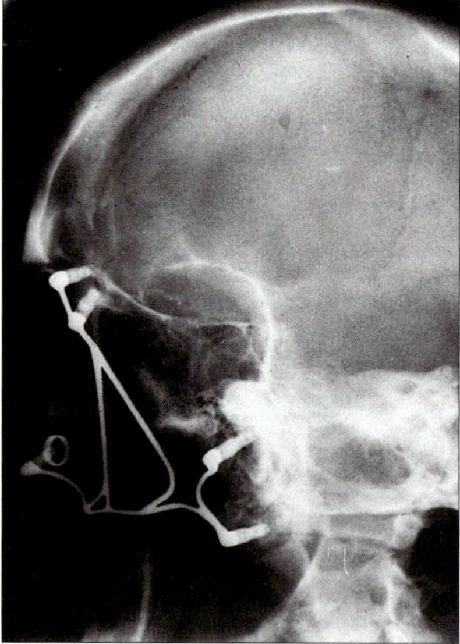

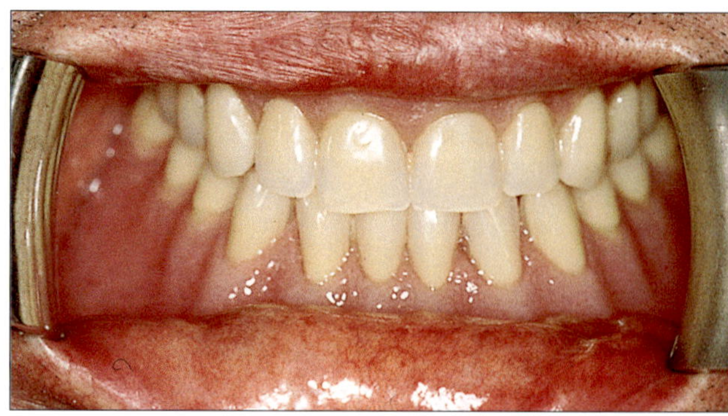

Fig 5-3g The framework and the relative positions of the fixtures can be seen in this radiograph.

Fig 5-3h The osseointegration technique allowed the rehabilitation team to provide this patient with a functioning set of teeth, which helped overcome his previous difficulty with eating.

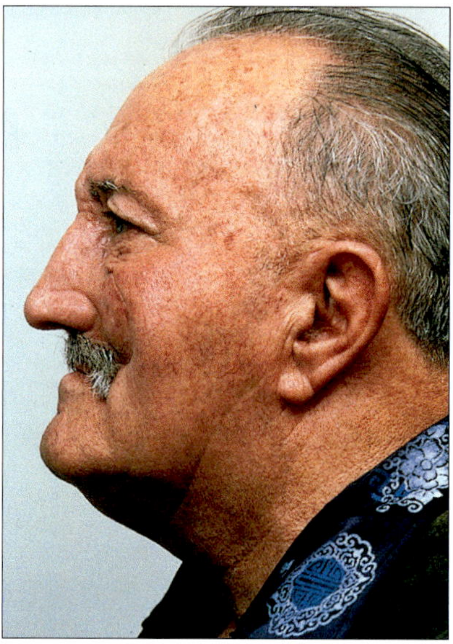

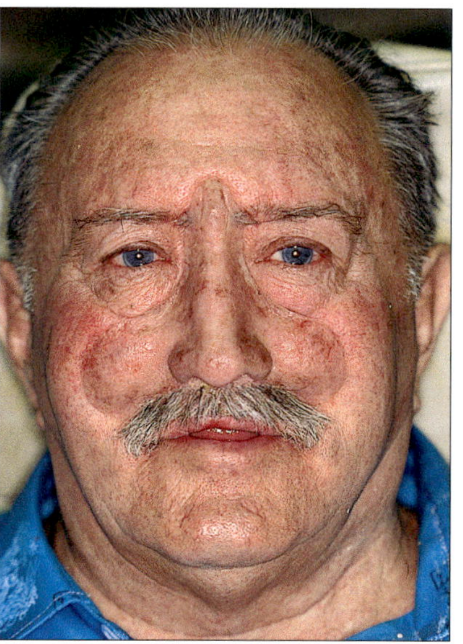

Figs 5-3i and **5-3j** The profile and full-face views of the patient once rehabilitation had been completed. The reconstruction work did not result in any complications. The treatment allowed him to live a normal life for many years.

have undergone earlier surgery with poor results or who cannot tolerate the plastic surgery procedure psychologically. Then, an ear prosthesis is an acceptable alternative. Normally such procedures are not recommended before a child is physically and emotionally mature enough to understand the choices and risks associated with any treatment. Often the clinician has to avoid the situation in which treatment is demanded by parents anxious to resolve their child's appearance problems as early as possible if it might jeopardize the success of future treatment modalities.

The Gothenburg team has considerable knowledge about the application of osseointegration to craniofacial situations. Though it was not until 1989 that the technique became more widely known via reports in the Swedish press, the team felt it could make some major improvements in its own rehabilitation program.

One aim was to reduce the time between radical surgery and the fitting of the prosthesis. Looking at cancer of the pinna, Anders Tjellström noted, "By the end of 1988, we had placed more than 750 implants in the mastoid and lost only 10. This success in terms of implant survival was one of the factors which encouraged us to start a trial with the one-stage surgical procedure." The team also knew that the force applied to a fixture by an ear prosthesis or a bone-anchored hearing aid, for example, was much less than that experienced by dental fixtures. Chewing forces were frequently 50 to 200 N and can reach peaks of 2,000 N while the axial force of a prosthesis weighing less than 50 g is estimated to be less than 1 N. Even the strain of attaching and removing the prosthesis is relatively low compared with the loading normally experienced in dental applications.

The single-stage procedure program started in February 1989 at Sahlgren's University Hospital. The study was restricted to the mastoid process and initially to only adult patients. By 1993, 161 patients had been treated according to this protocol. Eventually, the one-stage procedure began to be applied in other medical applications. This shows the importance of the interdisciplinary nature of the osseointegration work in allowing developments to flow between different applications and groups of patients.

6 Hearing and Being Heard

"Progress, therefore, is not an accident, but a necessity. ... It is part of nature."

Herbert Spencer, 1820-1903

Hearing impairment is a serious problem worldwide. Indeed, it is one of the most common forms of disability. There are a number of reasons for hearing loss, including congenital defects, infection, tumor, trauma, and aging. In the industrialized world alone, it has been estimated that approximately one-quarter of the population suffers from some degree of hearing loss, and this condition is often related to aging. Hearing impairment through aging is caused by loss of hair cells in the organ of Corti that results in a reduction in the ear's ability to pick up certain frequencies. Also, the eardrum and attached ossicles become more fixed and less able to transmit the mechanical sound waves. By the age of 50, about 20 percent of people have some degree of hearing impairment, with the figure rising to 50 percent at the age of 70 years.

Deafness is one of the most socially disabling conditions. Sufferers feel isolated and often withdraw from communication because of the difficulties and frustrations involved in interacting with others. In the infant and young child, deafness has even more striking consequences for social and intellectual participation.

While the deaf community has developed a rich communication culture through the medium of sign language, there continues to be a lively debate about when, how, or even, if, a child should be given treatment to restore or improve hearing. This debate is becoming increasingly important because of the emergence of new types of treatment that can overcome or alleviate a number of hearing defects.

Traditional Treatments

Any hearing aid is essentially an amplifier to boost the sound signal. It has four main components: a microphone to pick up the sound, an amplifier to intensify the sound signal, an earphone or transducer to deliver the sound to the ear, and a battery to provide the power. The majority of people with hearing problems that can be helped by a hearing aid are fitted with an air-conduction device that sits inside the ear canal. The technology and miniaturization of air-conduction devices, thanks to developments in electronics, means such devices offer a discreet solution for most common hearing difficulties. However, complications such as allergy, skin irritation, recurring infections in the auditory canal, or chronic inflammation of the middle ear can prevent the use of such devices.

At one time, the only alternative was to use a bone-conducting hearing aid in which the device has two transducers attached via a headband or spectacles pressed firmly against the skull. These are not inconspicuous designs. Such aids can be cumbersome and uncomfortable with variable improvement in overall hearing. They have to be pressed close to the side of the head to transmit sound through the layers of skin and bone. Sound energy is lost as it travels through tissue, and the higher frequencies tend to experience greater losses. The need to have a firm, constant pressure against the skull often causes its own problems for users, including pain, pressure sores, skin redness, and headaches.

Inner Ear Grafts and Bone-Anchored Hearing Aids

From the outset of his work in anchoring titanium components in bone, Per-Ingvar Brånemark and his colleagues realized there were many potential applications for the technique in most areas of the human frame. Indeed, the osseointegration work carried out in Gothenburg, Sweden, has led to a number of treatment regimes to restore or improve hearing. Professor Anders Tjellström, one of the prime researchers in this field, obtained his doctorate while working with Brånemark in the microcirculation laboratory. His work led to a new surgical technique for repairing hearing defects using autologous bone grafting.

The work was based on the development of a special mold, made from titanium, that could be inserted in a patient's tibia. This mold was intended to create a piece of bone shaped like the ossicle after a few months in situ. Once removed, this shaped bone could be grafted into the ear to replace a damaged or missing bone and restore hearing in suitable patients. In many ways, this was an adaptation of the osseointegration technique, as the titanium mold was not rejected by the bone and tissue during the period required to create the ossicle shape for subsequent transplantation.

Before this technique was developed, researchers had tried a number of alternative treatments using other types of bone materials, plastics, and metal. Such attempts had a relatively poor success rate in the long term, though continued efforts are underway. The autologous bone-graft technique carried out at Sahlgren's University Hospital's ear, nose, and throat (ENT) department has had continuing success.

In parallel with this work was the development of an approach with wider application potential – a new type of hearing system. Again this work was of a multidisciplinary nature, and Anders Tjellström and Olle Hallén of Sahlgren's University Hospital in Gothenburg provided surgical input. Richard Skalak, then at Columbia University in New York City, provided engineering expertise. Peder Carlsson and Bo Håkansson, at the Department of Applied Electronics, Chalmers Technical University in Gothenburg, led the devel-opment of the technical design of a new type of hearing aid called the bone-anchored hearing aid.

This device exploited the fact that humans hear in two ways. Sound vibrations, which are pressure waves, are picked up both by the ear canal and the temporal bone. These pressure waves set up mechanical vibrations in the inner ear by hitting the ear drum, a cone-shaped, translucent membrane. Other components in the inner ear – the anvil, stirrup, and hammer – act like amplifiers to intensify the tiny, but highly sensitive, movements of the ear drum. The resulting mechanical vibrations are transformed by the inner ear into electrical signals. Such signals are carried along the auditory nerve to the appropriate part of the brain for further processing and interpretation. The brain's sound processing system can identify approximately 350,000 discrete sounds. So rapid is the processing that identification can be completed within 0.03 seconds of the sound being picked up by the outer ear.

A number of researchers have looked at the potential of implant techniques to overcome these problems associated with traditional treatments. The osseointegration technique offers a more efficient way of providing bone-conductive hearing by allowing direct connection to the bone. The concept is to insert surgically a small titanium screw in the temporal bone behind the affected ear. Then a small, skin-penetrating abutment is used as an attachment point for a small hearing aid. As there is no sound-dampening effect from the skin, the aid can be small and hidden behind the ear. A bayonet coupling is the method by which the aid is connected and disconnected to the skin-penetrating abutment.

Bo Håkansson, an engineering researcher working at the Chalmers Technical University in Gothenburg, produced his doctoral thesis on an early form of this device in 1984. By this time, clinical studies were already underway and a limited number of patients had been treated. Håkansson suggested that a new hearing aid could be connected via a snap connector to the skin-penetrating abutment. Early designs had the transducer and microphone placed too close together, which resulted in acoustic feedback. These prototypes were quickly improved upon, and the first commercial design fit into a small rectangular box that fit neatly behind the ear.

Håkansson and another engineering colleague, Peder Carlsson, began to refine the design, taking advantage of the possibilities of further component miniaturization. Also, the two engineering researchers had worked closely with the ENT department at Sahlgren's University Hospital on the operations carried out on the first patients in 1977. It would take 11 years before the bone-anchored hearing aid was approved, in February 1988, by the Swedish National Social Welfare Board. After this it went into commercial development and was released onto the market. It was originally launched under the name Nobelpharma Auditory System HC200. Since then it has undergone refinement and further miniaturization and is now marketed by a company called Entific, which sells the system throughout the world.

Of course, there have been subtle refinements in the hearing system, but essentially the concept has remained unchanged since 1977. As Tjellström pointed out in 1999, "the flange fixture as designed by Brånemark and Viktor Kuikka in their workshop is exactly the same as [it was in] 1977. The design of the bone-anchored hearing aid used in association with osseointegration is essentially unchanged, which indicates the level of sound quality and performance that was achieved from the outset of the program."

Treating Children

One of the real challenges has been the treatment of children with congenital malformation, which can be combined with a hearing defect, usually both sensorineural and conductive loss. This type of hearing loss occurs in approximately 2 of every 1,000 cases. Premature babies suffer a higher incidence of hearing impairment, approximately 40 percent. As techniques improve to increase the survival rate of premature children, the issue of providing hearing solutions for this group becomes more imperative.

Different groups around the world are looking at the implications of providing children born with hearing defects with hearing aids as early as possible. Hearing within the first year of life is regarded as vital to the intellectual development and learning process. Children born with congenital atresia, but with normal cochlear function, can benefit intellectually and socially through the provision of a hearing aid as early as possible. In appropriate cases, cochlear implant surgery for the totally deaf child can be performed before the age of 6 months, Anders Tjellström has explained.

Children with normal cochlear function having congenital atresia can also benefit from the bone-anchored hearing aid. At Gothenburg's Carlander's Hospital, the ENT unit has fitted an 18-month-old child with such a device. In the United Kingdom at Birmingham's Queen Elizabeth Hospital, David Proops and his group have shown that providing children with hearing as early as possible allows them to acquire speech more fluently. The ability to produce distinct speech is reduced in hearing-impaired children when compared to those with a normal hearing capacity. When fitted with a bone-anchored hearing aid, the children are able to discriminate the high-frequency range of speech associated with the consonant sounds and so vital to the overall comprehension of speech. With the bone-anchored hearing aid, high frequencies are not lost in the soft tissue because there is direct bone conduction via an implant in the mastoid.

Other Developments

Another treatment regime that has been developed is to fit bilateral hearing aids. Though a single bone-anchored hearing aid can have a dramatic effect for the hearing impaired, some older patients have expressed the desire to gain more directional information through the provision of bilateral aids. A limited number of patients have been fitted with two bone-anchored hearing aids (Figs 6-1 to 6-4). To evaluate the benefits and effectiveness of bilateral aids, multicenter studies are being planned at centers in Gothenburg, Nijmegen in the Netherlands, Edmonton in Canada, Bauru in Brazil, and Birmingham in the United Kingdom.

Researchers believe that, for the bone-anchored hearing aid, efforts should continue to further improve sound quality and make the hearing aid as small as possible. In a 1999 thesis on bone conduction produced by Stefan Stenfeldt at Chalmers Technical University, he concluded that if the vibrations were introduced closer to the cochlea, sound distortions could be reduced. In addition, the transducer could be reduced in size and the overall quality of sound improved. This is possible because of the continued development of integrated electronics technology that packs more processing power into an ever-smaller space.

By early 2000, totally sealed implantable microphones having high sound quality were available and implantable rechargeable batteries were close to commercial reality. By the year 2005, Tjellström is convinced that clinical tests will be underway on totally implantable hearing aid technologies. Such concepts had been suggested both by Hallén and Skalak during the

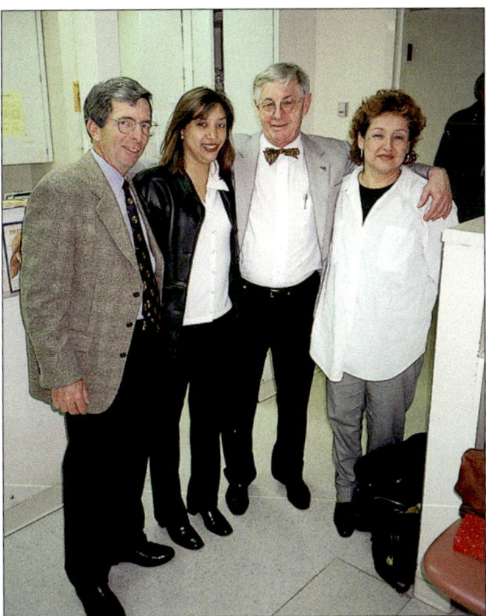

Fig 6-1 This patient from San Antonio, Texas, was born with Treacher Collins syndrome (second from left pictured with her prosthodontist, Professor Brånemark, and her mother). She had impaired hearing and microtia of both ears. Her treatment included the installation of bilateral fixtures for ear prostheses and bone-anchored hearing aids.

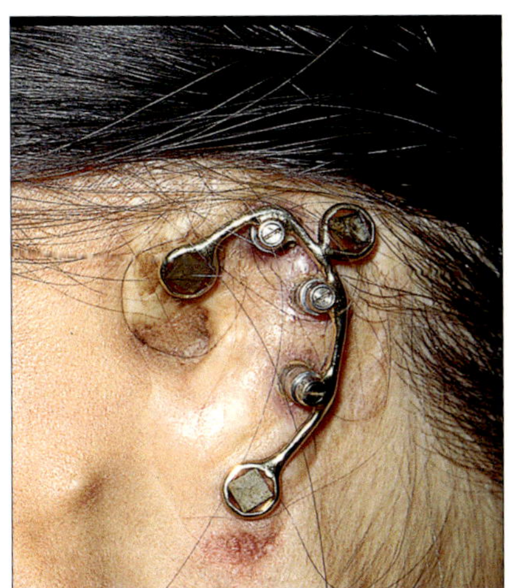

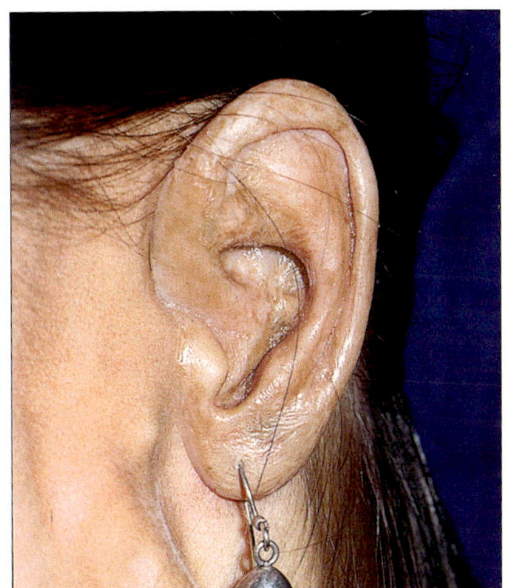

Figs 6-2a and **6-2b** Three fixtures from the anchorage points to which a frame is attached.

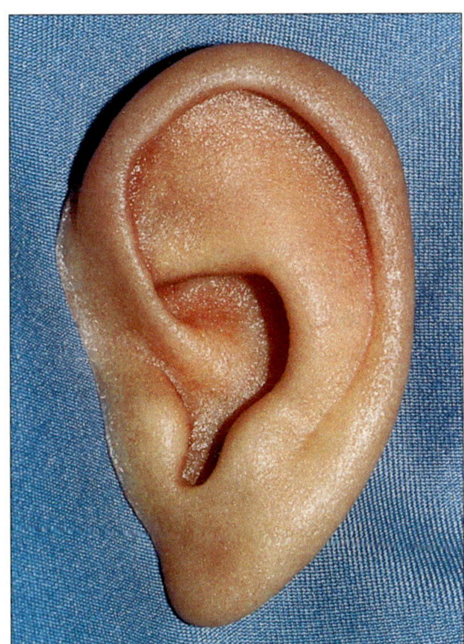

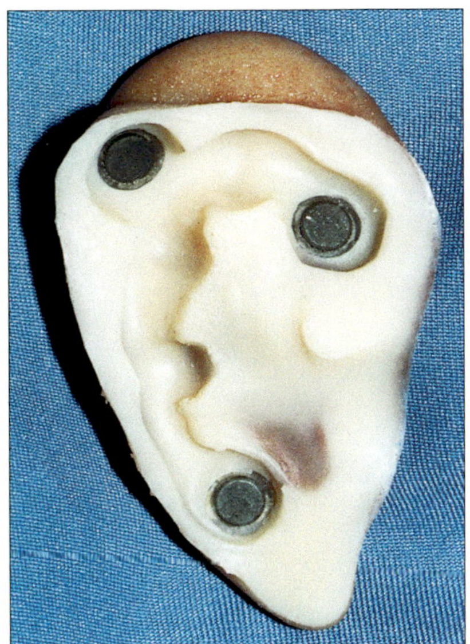

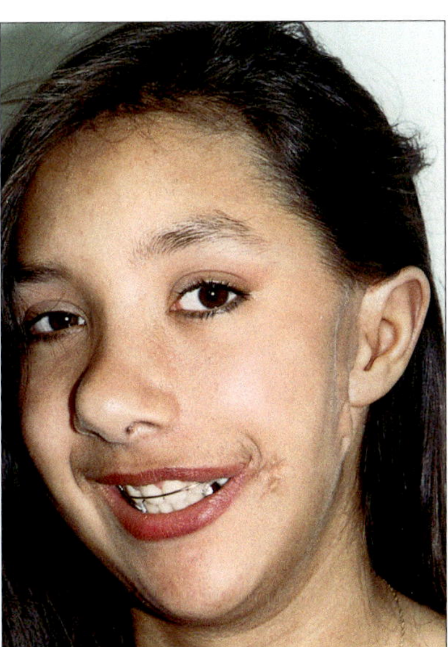

Figs 6-3a to **6-3c** The prosthetic ear clips to this frame using small magnets.

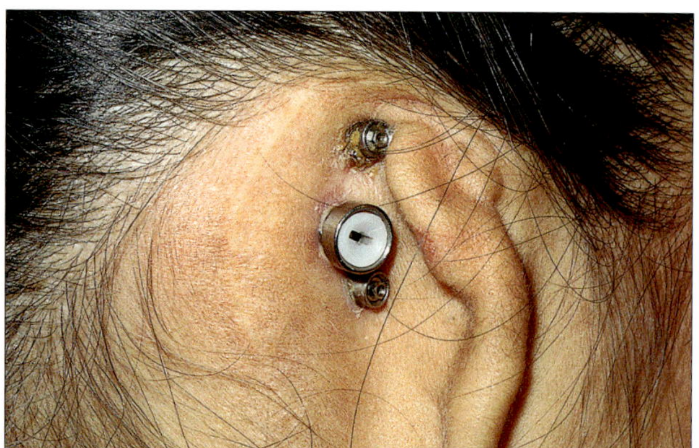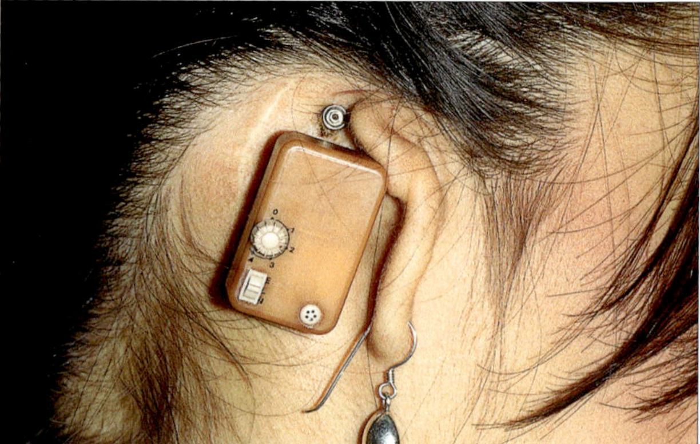

Figs 6-4a and **6-4b**   A single fixture provides the anchorage point for the bone-anchored hearing aid. The fixture has a bayonet fitting that allows the hearing aid to slide into position neatly behind the ear.

early years of research into the potential applications of osseointegration. Of course, the progress of such technologies is always dependent on how such treatment can be provided within a health care system and the availability of funds to pay for it.

7

A Delicate Touch

"The man who makes no mistakes does not usually make anything."
Edward John Phelps, 1822-1900

Hands are humans' most useful integrated tools. They can carry out delicate and intricate tasks, yet are capable of great strength. They support our facial expressions by conveying emotions and can even be used to communicate through a unique language for those unable to speak.

Our hands have a close relation to our brain, and through touch they are a vital medium for interpretation of our physical world. Children can learn the delights of cuddling soft toys, stroking furry animals, and squeezing gooey play materials, as well as the dangers of heat and sharp surfaces.

Losing the use of our hands, or even the hands themselves, strips us of the ability to carry out the most basic tasks. There are a number of reasons people can lose hand function. Humans, like other animals, are prey to a number of disorders affecting our joints. Rheumatoid arthritis is the most common cause of joint destruction in the hand and wrist. Osteoarthritis is the second most frequent cause of damage. Less common are tumors.

The consequences of these conditions are pain, coupled with loss of the ability to move joints, and varying degrees of deformation. These can have a devastating effect on the individuals concerned, making them dependent on others for assistance with dressing, eating, and moving objects.

When patients can no longer tolerate the constant pain or the incapacity of their situation, there is the option of artificial joint replacement. Often this surgical option is considered as a last resort when other types of therapy have failed.

In addition to joint disorders, some people lose their hands altogether. Trauma and birth defects are the main causes for the lack of or loss of the hand. In these cases it is not simply a matter of trying to recover loss of function but of offering a suitable artificial replacement for the hand and arm. Unlike the lower limbs, which are relatively straightforward to design, artificial arms and hands demand more intricate design considerations. For the lower limbs, the main considerations are support and the ability to take up the weight of the body during movement and at rest, as well as the ability to detect different types of surfaces. For the upper limbs, movement and sensibility are important design parameters because the hands are expected to complete far more complex tasks. The human hand is one of the most complex constructions within the human frame. Each contains 27 bones, which accounts for 13 percent of the total bones in the body.

Osseointegrative Solutions

Osseointegration is under development to provide both limb and joint replacement in the arms and hands. As mentioned previously, almost all the applications of osseointegration owe their origins in the fundamental research carried out in the microcirculation laboratory run by Per-Ingvar Brånemark from the early 1960s. As a skilled reconstructive surgeon, Brånemark believed osseointegration could have tremendous potential in the rehabilitation of patients suffering from a range of orthopedic problems related to conditions such as arthritis, trauma, or amputation.

Even some of the less-developed clinical applications today were mentioned or proposed more than a quarter of a century ago. This is true of the developments in applications involving the hand. One of the key figures in this respect is Göran Lundborg, a student of Brånemark's who gained his doctorate while working at the microcirculation laboratory in Gothenburg.

Lundborg's Work

Lundborg has always worked closely with the developments in osseointegration, although he has many other interests related to problems of the hand. In 1992, Lundborg was appointed as Sweden's only professor of hand surgery at Malmö General Hospital. He has a broad spectrum of work related to the repair and rehabilitation of patients with hand-related problems.

At a major conference on osseointegration, entitled "From Molecules to Man," held in 1999 in Gothenburg, Lundborg pointed out, "Though the ancestors of man had poorly developed brains, their hands were highly developed. Over time, the brain expanded because of the need to interpret the information gathered by the hand until in Homo sapiens, the brain has reached its current capacity. This has made other mental functions possible such as verbal capacity, for example."

Stereognosis allows humans the ability to identify shapes, delicate textures, and structures. Working in harmony with the brain, the hand allows humans to recognize, remember, and identify specific items. The sense of touch is such a powerful and useful sense that it can be used to replace other senses. Lundborg explains that this is possible because of several types of sensory receptors in the glabrous skin of our fingertips and free nerve endings in the epidermal layers. These pick up nerve signals transmitted via nerve fibers in the nerve trunks to their final destination in the somatosensory brain cortex where specific projectional areas representing each digit are located (Fig 7-1).

The hand and the face together occupy major parts of the sensory cortex. The adult brain continually remaps its own functional contour. Sensory maps can be redrawn and remodeled in a feature termed brain plasticity. This functional brain remodeling process is activity-dependent and based on weakening or strengthening synaptic functions in the brain. For example, in primate studies it was found that if a finger is specifically trained in a sensory task, the cortical territory representing this digit expands. The digit takes over new cortical territories, and the receptive fields in the tips of the fingers become very small, resulting in improved tactile acuity.

In humans, the finger used by a blind person to read Braille has an increased cortical representation. Violin players practicing 6 to 8 hours per day also have an increased cortical representation of the fingers of the left fingering hand. Thus the brain assigns or maps itself ac-

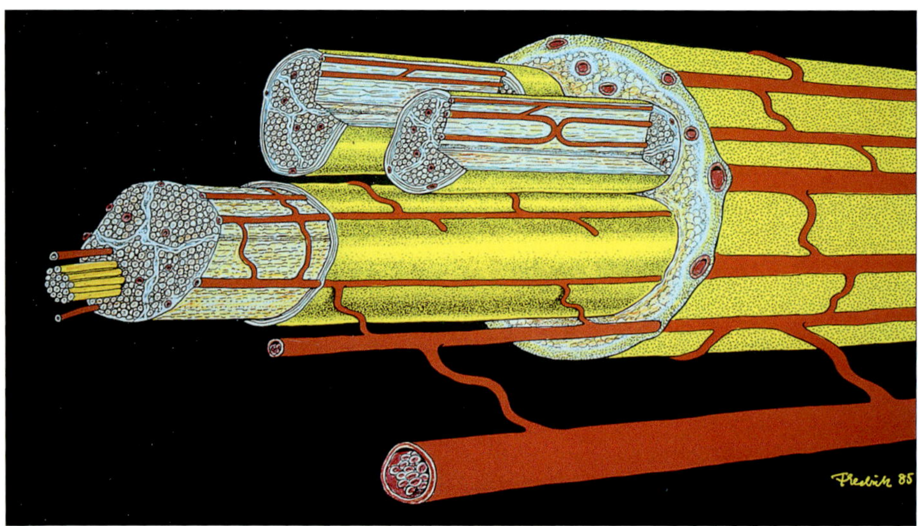

Fig 7-1 The microvascular patterns of nerves.

cording to the information it receives from physical sensors.

In reconstructive surgery, a so-called sleeping sensibility can be reawakened and improved stereognosis achieved. This has been noted following procedures where the contracted hand of a patient with cerebral palsy is opened up using tendon transfers, exposing the palm of the hand to tactile experiences.

Exposure to excess sensory stimuli can also provoke a negative response as exemplified by repetitive, monotonous, non-physiological movement typical of extensive keyboard use. In some cases, ystonia, an inability to coordinate, may occur. In what has been classed as repetitive strain injury (RSI), the pain may be in the brain. In similar cases in primates, normal hand representation is severely deranged, and the sensory map of the hand is totally changed. Receptive fields in the fingertips are enlarged considerably. This means that a touch anywhere in the hand can excite the same cortical neurons.

In nerve injuries, the nerve can be repaired. In the brain, the sensory cortex responds to the injury by loss of representation of the damaged parts of the hand. The bands that represent the denervated skin area are replaced, literally, by a black hole in the corresponding area because of the acute deafferentiation or loss of sensory input. Soon, however, the adjacent areas of the cortex rapidly take over the empty area. After axonal outgrowth, unfortunately often to the wrong destinations in the hand, there is total remodeling of the brain cortex. In some respects this is rather like the hand speaking a new language to the brain, which the mind can no longer interpret. To overcome this, re-education is required to reprogram the brain and regain functional sensibility by feeling, looking, concentrating, and feeling again, just as the newborn child experiences and learns from its new environment.

Lundborg and his co-workers have been interested in how this knowledge can be used to help in hand rehabilitation and also how it could be applied in the development of treatment regimes to improve the outcome for patients. This includes osseointegration to improve the function of implant designs. The interaction of the hand and the brain is proving to be a fertile ground for exploration, and there is still much to learn. In parallel with this work, there is still progress to be made on basic joint mechanisms to improve existing artificial limb designs.

Prosthetic Joints

All joints are constructed in a similar way, as their purpose is to hold our bones together and allow movement between bones. They are classified into three types according to the amount of freedom of movement they allow. Those that allow the greatest amount of movement, diarthroses, consist of a joint capsule, a joint cavity, and a layer of cartilage that spans the ends of two bones. The joint capsule is constructed from the body's strongest and toughest material called fibrous connective tissue. This is lined with smooth, slippery synovial membrane. The capsule fits over the ends of the two bones like a sleeve. The diarthroses are classed according to the type of movement they provide: ball and socket joints in the hips and shoulders, saddle joints in the thumb, and hinge joints in the fingers and knees.

Artificial joint designs that can mirror exactly the operation of healthy human joints are extremely difficult to achieve. There are many factors to consider: the mechanics of the joint, the anchorage of the implant to the bone, the interaction of the human tissues and the implant, anticipated loading and wear, and the particular properties of the implant material.

Today medical researchers have a rich source of materials from which to create implant components, including plastics, metals, and ceramics. Attempts have been going on for almost 90 years to create working artificial joints for the fingers and wrist. By the 1950s, joint replacement research led to the development of metallic hinged devices that were largely unsuccessful because of metallic corrosion, skin breakdown, bone resorption, and a poor restoration of movement. By the 1970s, a range of different designs appeared using a combination of metal and plastic fixed by bone cement. Sadly, most of these devices never lived up to their inventors' hopes, and few finger designs have survived today.

One of the most widely used solutions to finger-joint replacements are those made of silicone elastomer. Silicone is regarded as a very suitable material for implant purposes. Apart from its low cost, it has good flexing characteristics, durability, heat stability, and load dampening properties. There are disadvantages, however. Any tear in the material can quickly travel through the silicone, causing a catastrophic failure. Two silicone finger-joint replacement designs were developed independently by Alfred Swanson and J.J. Niebauer. Swanson's simple design still remains one of the most widely used. It is a solid piece of silicone that is cone shaped at both ends. The two pointed ends of the artificial joint fit into the hollow bone marrow in the center of the bones. This single piece of plastic provides a simple solution and can give acceptable cosmetic results and provide pain relief. Some function is restored, although over the long term the implant can fracture, and sometimes there is an adverse body function with gradual worsening of the movement in the joint. All other types of finger-joint replacement mechanisms exhibit similar problems to a greater or lesser degree.

The imperfection of current finger-joint designs has prompted Lundborg and Brånemark to continue their efforts to create a better design based on osseointegration. There is no obvious reason why such a design should not be successful. However, providing a long-term solution based on osseointegration is proving to be a challenge. A design developed in the 1980s based on osseointegration uses two titanium screws and a silicone spacer. The titanium screws are inserted into each end of the finger joint and the spacer forms the moving joint component. Only the titanium is in direct contact with the bone. Theoretically, the rubbing and wear problems associated with other silicone-based solutions are avoided (Fig 7-2).

Clinical Studies

Clinical studies on this design began in 1980 and 1981 with the first groups of patients. Between 1988 and 1994, 150 metacarophalangeal joints were operated on in 45 hands (accounting for 38 patients). The age range of patients was wide – from 22 to 74 years old. Most patients were suffering from rheumatoid arthritis, though several hands had been damaged by primary osteoarthrosis, post-traumatic osteoarthrosis, and post-infectious osteoarthrosis. By 1997, the longest follow-up period was 6 years and the patients' hand function was evaluated according to their ability to carry out various tasks.

The surgical procedure for the insertion of osseointegrated finger joints was carried out under general anesthesia and initially followed the protocols prescribed by Swanson. Over each joint a dorso-ulnar longitudinal incision was made. The extensor hood was incised to the ulnar side of

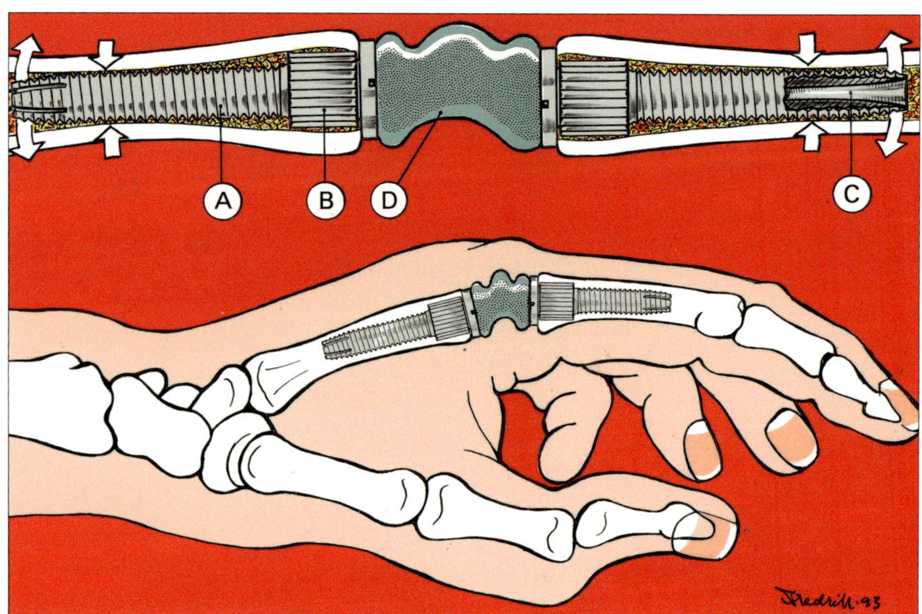

Fig 7-2 The original concept for a finger-joint replacement developed in the 1980s based on osseointegration. This uses two titanium screws (A) and a silicone spacer (D). The titanium screws are inserted into each end of the finger joint, and the spacer forms the moving joint component. (B) Connection piece. (C) The tapered ends of the fixture fit along the length of the bone cavity.

the extensor tendon, and appropriate amounts of the metacarpal heads were resected. Then, longitudinal cylindrical channels were carefully drilled by hand into the medullary cavities of the metacarpal and phalangeal bones. As for all osseointegration procedures, extreme care was taken to ensure that heat was not generated to damage the bone, hence the use of hand drills.

It is usual that rheumatoid patients present with fatty, loosely textured marrow and the diaphysis has thin, dense, and brittle cortical bone. In such cases, the marrow cavities were always packed with grafts of cancellous bone and marrow from the iliac crest. The titanium screws were then carefully secured in the previously drilled holes of the metacarpal and phalangeal bones. Also, before the fixtures were introduced into the bone, their surface was covered by autogenous marrow blood from the patient. This was applied to support the body's natural healing process. A silicone spacer was attached to the titanium screws by providing a short titanium stem from the spacer to the central channel in the screw. One of the key aspects of this design is the fact that a spacer can be replaced at a later date without affecting the osseointegration process.

At the time these procedures were being developed, the surgical team was faced with a particular challenge. It had been considered that for osseointegration to be successful, the underlying bone with its titanium components needed to be unloaded and undisturbed to give time for the integration to take place. In dental applications, this was easy to achieve. In arthritis sufferers, joints tend to become stiff and painful, and patients need to continue to exercise to preserve what limited movement they have. Lundborg devised a gentle postoperative exercise plan for patients, which was sufficient to maintain movement without jeopardizing the osseointegration process. This rehabilitation regime starts on the fifth postoperative day. It is carried out under the supervision of an experienced hand therapist and involves controlled movements using dynamic splints. Full range of motion and light functional activities without splints were suggested by the sixth week postoperatively, with moderate to heavy activities not encouraged until 3 months after surgery.

The evaluation work on this relatively small number of cases found that osseointegration oc-curred in practically all cases, even though the implant was loaded after the fifth postoperative day. These patients were often on fairly heavy medication because of their conditions. Most of the patients, for example, were receiving permanent steroid or cytotoxin medication for the treatment of their basic disease.

By 1997, results of a detailed follow-up of the group's first 68 patients were presented based on an average follow-up of 2.5 years (ranging from 6 to 54 months). In rheumatoid patients, the average range of motion was 57 degrees, and it was 50 degrees for all cases. Osseointegration was successful in all cases, though there was a fracture of the spacer in 6 percent of patients.

The fact that osseointegration was successful for most patients eventually led Brånemark and his co-workers to reconsider loading factors in other clinical areas. Indeed, this has contributed to the development of the single-stage surgery and the same-day teeth concept. Immediate loading is possible, providing it is beneficial, or at least neutral, to the osseointegration process. The interdisciplinary nature of the work lends itself to this cross fertilization of ideas so many areas can benefit from progress or new information discovered by other teams.

Treating Arthritis

The potential to help arthritis sufferers who are beyond any further conventional medical intervention is enormous. Arthritis is a very distressing disease that affects many millions worldwide, of which a small but still significant number are extremely disabled by the condition. Caring for such sufferers coupled with the cost of medication to provide pain relief is an enormous drain financially.

While the results from Sweden had been encouraging, other teams in Australia had attempted to replicate them but had not achieved similar positive results. This proved a considerable disappointment and consequently the finger-joint prosthesis still remains a long way from commercial reality. While the osseointegration of the titanium components is highly successful, the spacer mechanism has proved to be the major stumbling block. The main aim of recent work has been to reduce the failure level in this intermediate but vital component. The re-

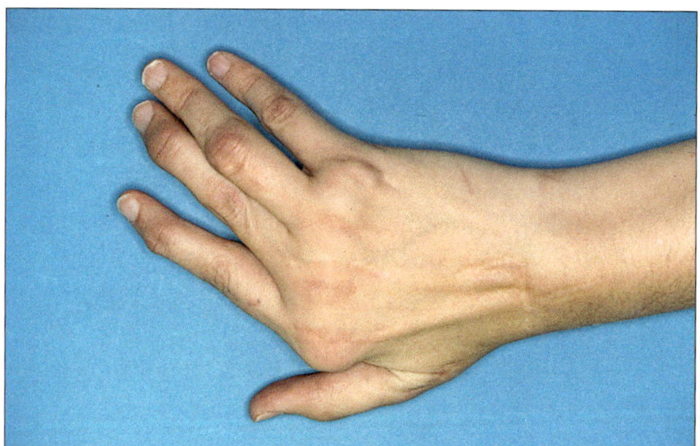

Fig 7-3a Prior to treatment, this patient's hand shows the damage caused by rheumatoid arthritis. The typical deformation of the hand results in constant pain, plus difficulty in movement and control.

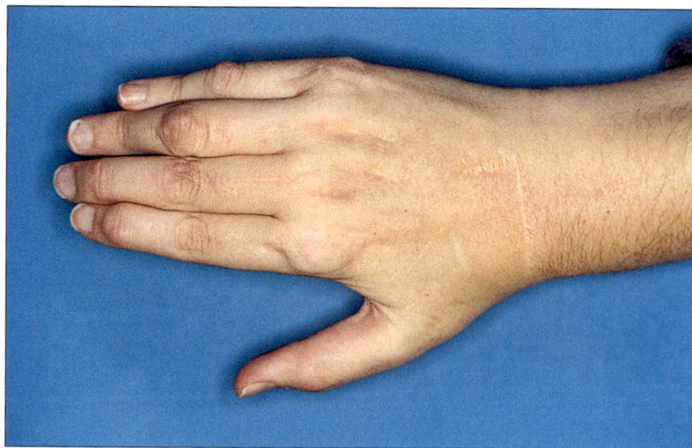

Fig 7-3b Following finger-joint replacement procedures using osseointegration, the same rheumatic hand has a more normal appearance. The range of function has also been considerably restored, allowing the patient to carry out normal daily tasks.

searchers have been trying to establish why the silicone spacer design has a tendency to fail, and they have tried to find a better solution to this key component in the finger joint. Recently new materials have been tried on a number of patients, and the preliminary results have been extremely encouraging. Hopefully longer-term follow-up will confirm the improvements (Figs 7-3a and 7-3b).

Brånemark points out that it is important to learn lessons from each case, especially those regarded as failures. Until a better joint mechanism is found, the team will be cautious about the type of surgical procedures carried out relating to finger-joints. Finger-joint patients treated with the osseointegration procedure will be carefully monitored, and the knowledge gained from these cases will be used to build the information base about osseointegration in hand applications. Lundborg and his co-workers believe the main efforts now going into the development of improved materials will eventually achieve the right combination of mechanical strength, biocompatibility, and mobility.

One positive aspect of the work is that in rheumatoid arthritis sufferers, osseointegration treatment has involved using the patient's own marrow at the implant site, which Brånemark has always been convinced helps promote bone healing. In light of information gained about the role of stem cells and other components of marrow in new growth, this has been proved correct. In rheumatoid arthritis sufferers treated,

there has been no recurrence of the disease postoperatively, and the introduction of marrow during the procedures is believed to play a key role in this.

Hand and Arm Applications of Osseointegration

The use of osseointegration in other hand and arm applications has had far more immediate success. However, prosthetic alternatives in the hand and arm represent a number of challenges because of the complexity of the tasks these parts perform.

The osseointegration work has been clinically applied to a variety of simple and complex prosthetic applications in these parts of the body. The first patient treated in this region in 1990 was a 40-year-old male who had lost all the fingers of one hand, plus half of the palm, in an industrial accident. The effect of the accident, apart from the physical damage caused, was long-term depression and an inability to continue working. The possibility of early retirement was considered for this patient prior to the offer of rehabilitation using osseointegration methods. Titanium components were placed in the residual portion of the hand and a prosthesis was designed to allow the patient to grip and hold things. The results were very positive, and after treatment the patient was able to return to full-time work performing light duties.

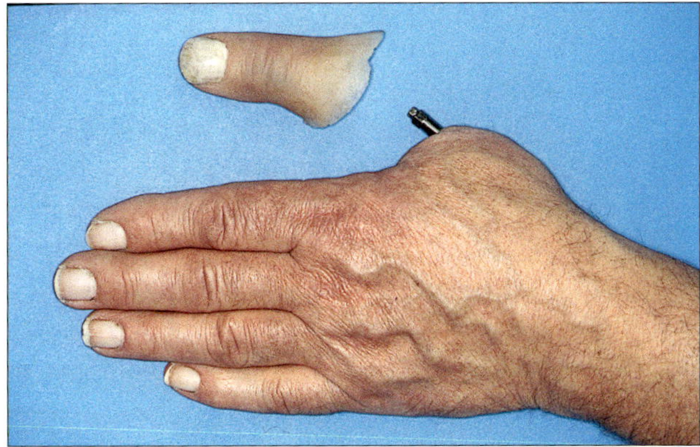

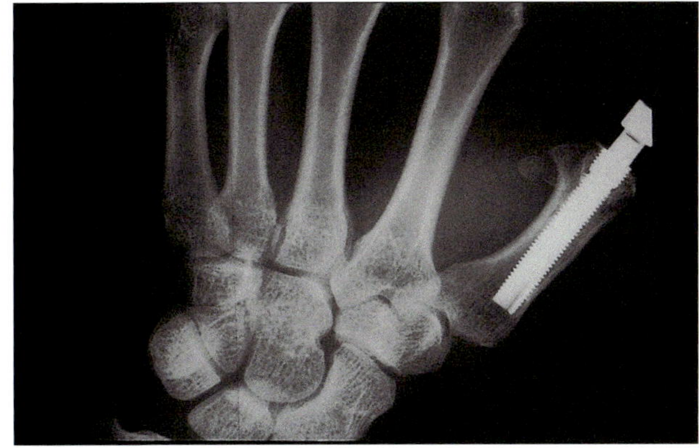

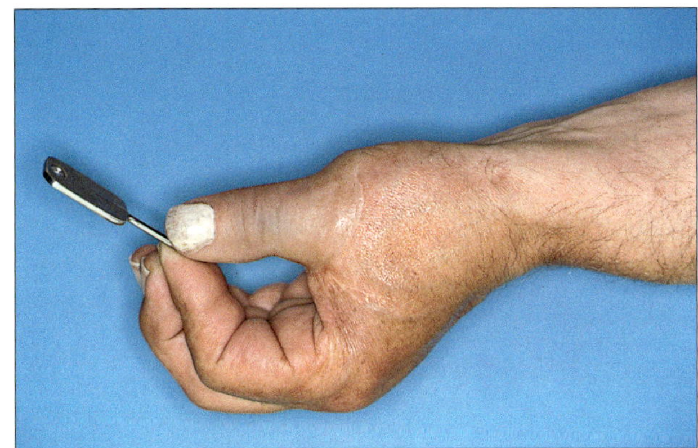

Figs 7-4a to **7-4c** A thumb prosthesis can be attached by the insertion of a fixture in the residual bone. This allows the patient to grip and even sense objects.

The range of patients with upper limb loss treated has been quite broad. For example, the team has developed a simple but effective prosthetic thumb design (Figs 7-4a to 7-4c). This is an alternative to the surgical procedure of using a patient's big toe as a thumb. One of the first patients to undergo this prosthetic procedure was Sven Persson. On September 25, 1990, Persson, a crane operator, was working on a crane some 13 m in the air. While making some adjustments to the crane, he had an accident that resulted in the loss of his whole thumb. The doctors tried to reattach the thumb, but the operation could not restore function so it had to be removed again. Persson had also lost the feeling in his other fingers in that hand.

In 1991 he had a titanium fixture implanted as a means of attaching a prosthetic thumb. He could have chosen to lose a toe and have that replace the lost thumb. However, he was reluctant to have such an operation. Persson commented of the prosthetic procedure, "I wanted to try it. If it did not work I could always have it removed." However, removal of his toe was not necessary, as the prosthesis has functioned well.

In 1994, he had to have the abutment changed because it had come loose. He has a number of thumb prostheses, which he changes depending on the type of activity he is carrying out. His work thumb is made from a harder material to cope with his daily work. As a result of the rehabilitation, Persson was able to return to work as a crane driver.

An example of a more complex procedure is the case of Eric Ulander. Born in 1934, Ulander trained as a mechanical engineer and spent many years working in the paper industry. On December 7, 1977, while changing the felt on the rollers of the paper machine, he had a horrific accident that resulted in the loss of both hands and damage to his arms. "A very dangerous situation arose, and I didn't realize before I was caught in the machine. I was wearing working gloves. These had high friction. I couldn't get out of the gloves. I was close to being killed. No one knew. My colleague was on the other side of the machine."

These machines are 30 feet wide and operate in a very noisy environment. When Ulander's colleague saw what was happening, he pressed

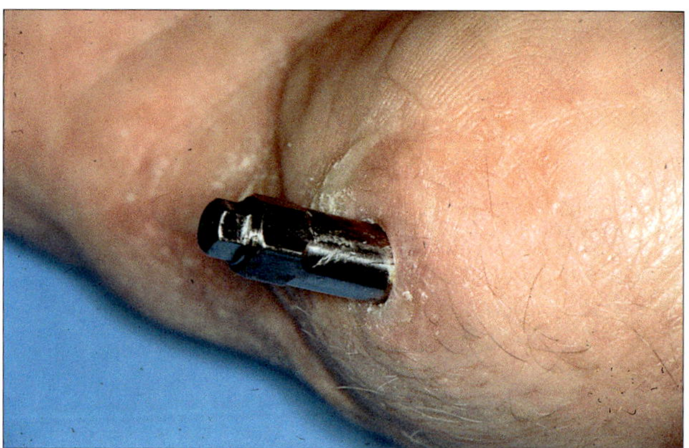

Fig 7-5 For upper limb amputees, skin-penetrating abutments are used. These provide an external anchorage point for hand or arm prostheses. This can help avoid skin irritation and other problems.

the stop button on the machine. Ulander was stuck in the machine for 2 or 3 minutes, but he was able to argue with colleagues about the best way of getting him out of the machine. He was fully conscious and not in that much pain. He said he felt in great spirits because he knew he had survived. He was rushed to the hospital and treated, but he required extensive rehabilitation.

At that time, the treatment available involved only conventional prosthetics coupled with some surgical intervention, including skin grafting. The surgeons tried to save as much as possible of both arms. On the right side, the right elbow was preserved but on the left side, it was not possible to retain this joint. By May 1980, Ulander was back to full-time work with the same company with two upper limb prostheses to meet his needs. At work, he moved into development projects. This turned out to be very suitable for the next decade or so, as he was able to use his experience internationally.

From about 1980, quite early in his rehabilitation, Ulander suffered bouts of inflammation and infection of the skin caused by the use of conventional prosthetic limbs in which his residual limbs fit into a socket attachment. Though he used creams, the chronic nature of the infection meant that he had to have a number of operations on the surrounding skin, and he was unable to wear the prostheses for long periods of time. He jokes that he felt he would soon run out of skin. As a result of these severe tissue problems, Ulander became one of the first candidates for the osseointegration implant technique as it became available.

The first of a series of operations for Ulander took place on June 29, 1993, with the new type of prosthesis attached in September 1993. Eventually, both arms were provided with osseointegrated implants to provide connection points for prostheses. As is usually the case for complex osseointegration procedures, the addition of autologous marrow blood from the patients is used to cover the surface before fixtures are introduced to residual bone. Not only was the infection problem alleviated but there have been other benefits. "I can feel direct contact with the prosthesis," noted Ulander. This gave him better control of movement and even a measure of sensitivity lacking with conventional artificial limbs. He demonstrated this by showing how he could pick up eggs without breaking them. Also, the simpler method of attachment gave him a greater degree of movement than before (Fig 7-5).

Ulander quickly became used to wearing his new prostheses. In particular, he found he had greater freedom of movement with his right hand side than he had before. He is able to raise his prosthesis on this side above his head, something that would not have been possible before because of the constrictions imposed by the conventional prosthetic arm designs. Being an engineer, Ulander was able to provide useful comments about his situation, and this information has been valuable in the further design of the attachment. Such pioneering patients are considered a key part of the team, and their concerns and comments are an important part of the development and evaluation process.

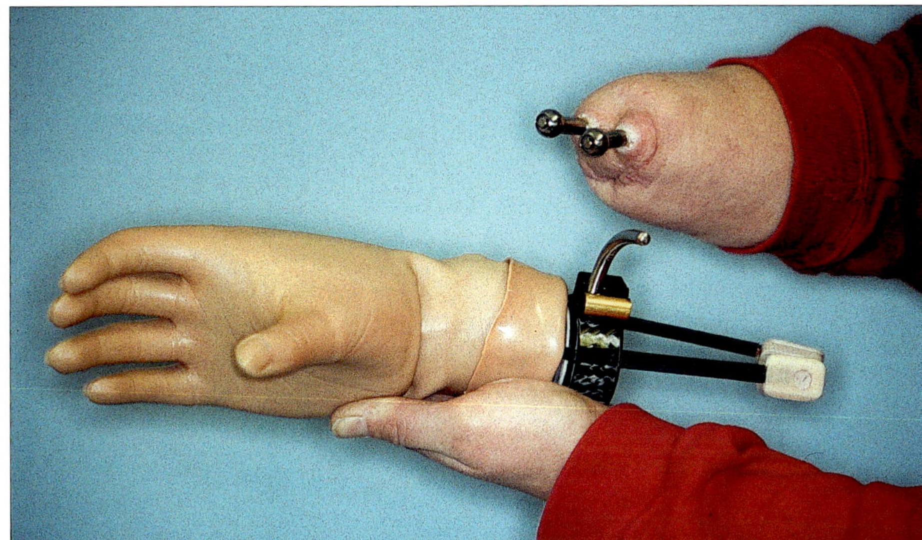

Fig 7-6 This patient's hand prosthesis is attached by two skin-penetrating abutments and has a conventional myo-electric connection.

Special Fixtures

For hand and arm prostheses, it is usual to provide two specially designed fixtures. Conventional myoelectric connection can also be used in conjunction with the hand prosthesis to provide the sensing mechanism for movement control (Fig 7-6).

Esthetic results for hand prostheses can be extremely life-like with the added benefit that the connection mechanism is less cumbersome than traditional designs (Fig 7-7).

One patient has had electrodes implanted into muscles with the aim of improving the function of an upper-body prosthesis (Figs 7-8a and 7-8b). The electrodes are attached via a separate implanted abutment, while two large skin-penetrating abutments provide the main connection for the prosthesis. So far, the follow-up period for implanted electrodes has been 5 years, and the experience gained with this patient will provide key information for further development. Brånemark notes, "A bone-anchored lower arm or hand prosthesis as well as a lower limb prosthesis might enable, because of mechanical stability and perception through brain controlled 'relais,' considerable improvement of the movements of the prosthetic limb."

In the future it may be possible to combine osseointegrated components with more sophisticated electronic control systems to restore the full range of natural movements and function to patients, whatever their disability.

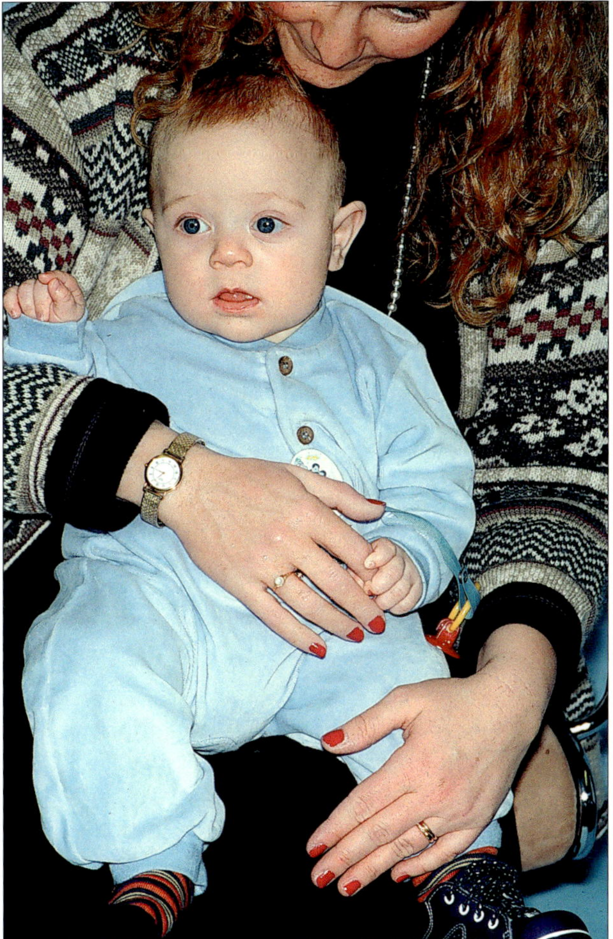

Fig 7-7 The esthetic results for this patient's hand prosthesis are extremely life like.

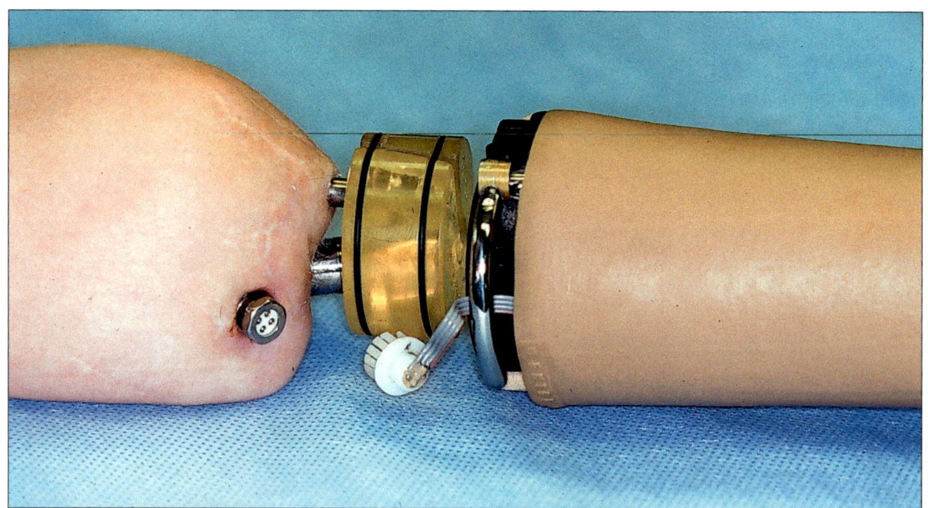

Fig 7-8a This patient has an implanted electrode system to replace the conventional myo-electric connection.

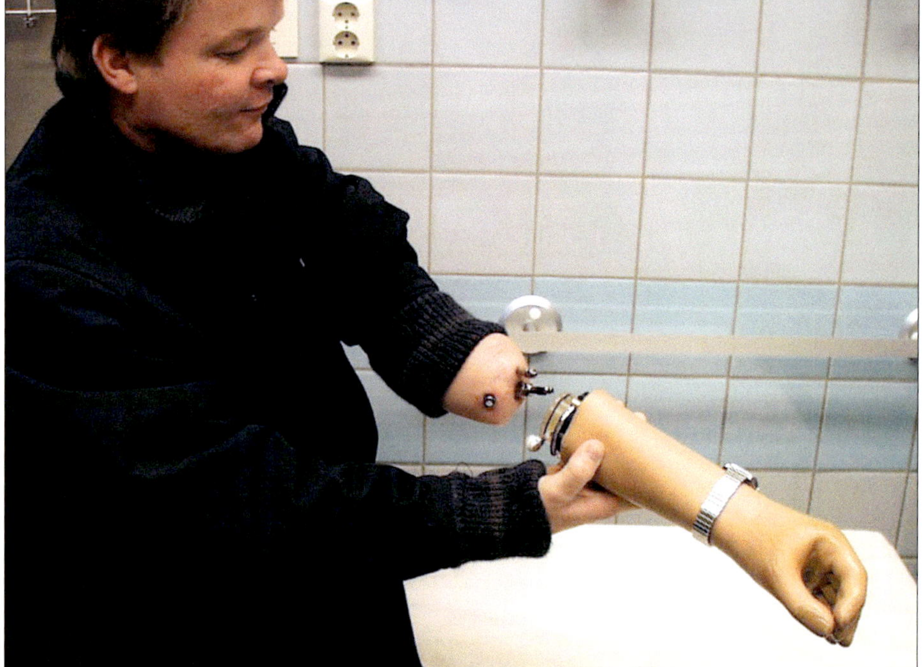

Fig 7-8b The addition of the implanted electrode means the connection of a hand or arm prosthesis is greatly simplified compared to traditional prosthetic solutions.

8

Solid Ground

"Desperate diseases require desperate remedies."
Guy Fawkes, 1570-1606

In parallel with the upper limb, hand, and joint work, Per-Ingvar Brånemark had always been interested in the possibility of using osseointegration for the whole range of orthopedic applications, in part because of his extensive experience in reconstructive surgery. The lower limbs present no less a challenge in terms of providing adequate function combined with an esthetically appropriate result (Fig 8-1). Today, artificial designs for lower limbs tend to be rather primitive and have a number of drawbacks for users.

The reasons why people need artificial limbs vary. In the industrialized world, the main reasons for lower limb amputation are related to peripheral vascular disease, including atherosclerosis and diabetic microangiopathy (Fig 8-2). Together these account for 85 to 90 percent of all lower limb amputations. Trauma accounts for 5 to 8 percent of cases, with tumors the cause of approximately 4 to 6 percent of cases, and the remaining 1 to 2 percent the result of infection or congenital malformations. In many other countries, the loss of lower limbs is related to injuries caused by land mines left buried following major conflicts. It has been estimated that 100 million land mines still litter our planet, presenting a hidden and ever-present danger.

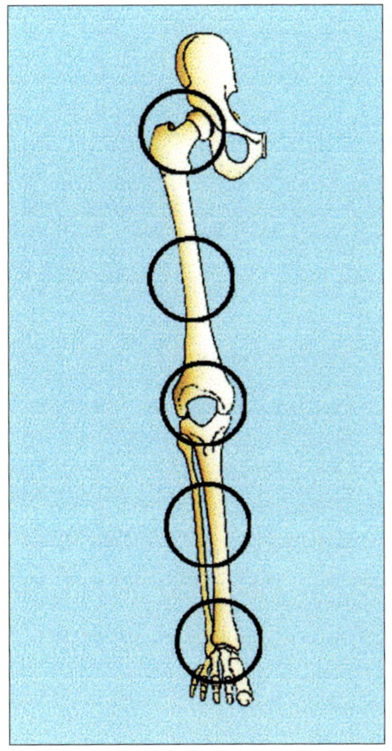

Fig 8-1 Regions in the lower limb where clinical applications involving osseointegration procedures are being developed or are already a reality.

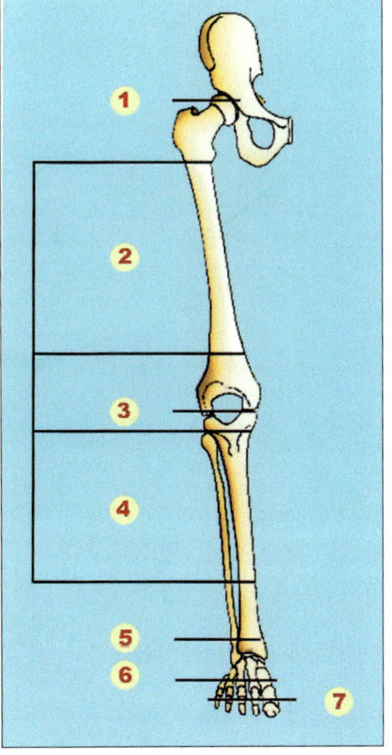

Fig 8-2 Amputation levels of the lower extremity. (1) Hip disarticulation; (2) above-knee amputation; (3) knee disarticulation; (4) below-knee amputation; (5) Syme's amputation; (6) transmetatarsal amputation; (7) toe amputation.

Current Treatments

Under ideal conditions, the surgeon carrying out the amputation attempts to provide an optimal stump length for any subsequent prosthesis. Textbooks provide guidelines for the various amputations, but an optimal situation is not always possible. This can be due to post-traumatic deformities or tumor resection surgery. The compromises made have consequences for the "socket" prosthesis. Without an adequate stump, the device may not perform entirely satisfactorily.

Even those with optimal residual stumps cannot be guaranteed problem-free prostheses. Skin infections and ulcerations frequently occur. Subcutaneous tissue and muscles may atrophy, which can lead to the need for frequent change of the prosthesis. Stump pain may be an additional problem, sometimes as the result of nerve compression, or neuroma. In other patients, inexact motor control may be another problem. Some patients find that ill-fitting prosthetic designs and changes that can occur with their stump over time mean artificial limbs become impossible to wear.

The time and cost of providing a patient with a properly fitting, conventional artificial limb can be extensive. One patient commented that he had six useless limbs in the cupboard and was wheelchair bound because none of the designs were suitable. Orthopedic engineers have calculated that for amputee patients with such problems, the total cost of treatment would be considerably reduced if osseointegration could be used as an anchorage.

Implementing Osseointegration

There are a number of opportunities to use osseointegration in the lower limbs, including joint and limb replacements. The work on orthopedic applications was initiated at the Institute for Applied Biotechnology and the Brånemark Osseointegration Center in collaboration with the Sahlgren's University Hospital in Gothenburg and other institutes (Fig 8-3).

Clinical work on an osseointegrated artificial lower limb began in 1990, although, to a significant degree, the technique was derived from the experiences of dental reconstruction and transcutaneous osseointegrated titanium implants in the head and neck. Providing an anchorage point for large artificial limbs is not a trivial issue, as the distribution of load and stresses becomes a major concern.

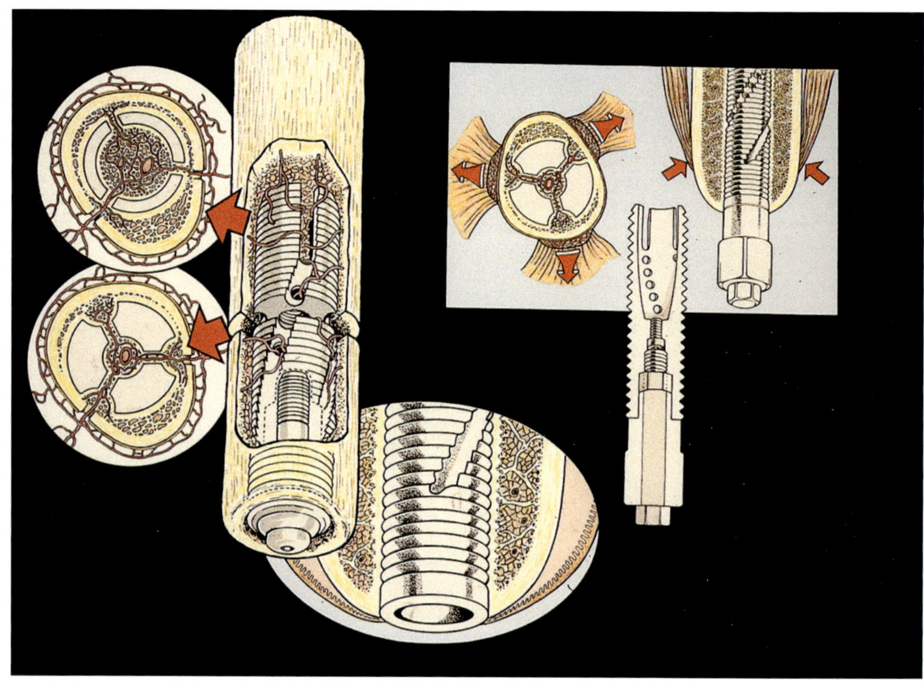

Fig 8-3 Concept behind skin-penetrating fixtures suitable for the attachment of limb prostheses.

It was a letter from a young patient, Teija Nilsson, that moved Brånemark to take a more active role in providing a solution for those who had lost limbs through trauma or cancer. As had been the case in the original dental work, Brånemark and the team were determined that their initial goal would be to help those patients whose difficulties were such that conventional treatment could not provide an immediate solution to their problems.

Nilsson became the first person to receive an osseointegrated attachment for the connection of an artificial limb. Her story is an unusual one. At 14 years old, in 1980, she had been the victim of a tram accident that resulted in the loss of both legs. The nature and extent of her injuries left her wheelchair bound with little hope using conventional artificial legs. Two years after her accident, Nilsson read an article about Brånemark's work, which mentioned that the titanium screws, once integrated into bone, were so strong they could support a load of up to 50 kg. This set the teenager thinking, "I weighed only 45 kg, so why couldn't it be used for me?" She contacted Brånemark's clinic, and this was the start of a long-term relationship with the professor.

As an experienced reconstructive surgeon, Brånemark was well aware of the potential osseointegration offered in this regard. However, there were a number of technical problems and practical issues to overcome before it could reach clinical reality. This included the development of a method to directly connect a prosthetic limb to the osseointegrated fixture and a redesign of the artificial limb to accommodate the osseointegrated component. Also the biomechanical implications of different types of loading on the fixture, residual bone, and tissue had to be considered to provide a suitably fail-safe design.

Brånemark felt it was important to solve most of the questions surrounding these issues before embarking on any clinical work. This required the collaboration of a wide range of specialists in mechanics, surgery, prosthetic design, etc. The clinical procedure would be similar to that used in dental applications. The fixture used would be a giant version of the tiny dental fixtures, and new prosthetic limb attachments would be created.

Nilsson's case was extremely challenging. Conventional prosthetic rehabilitation was not an option, owning to the shortness of her residual limbs. Brånemark felt that if a solution could be found for this patient, it might be applied successfully to less difficult cases.

Though the lower limb is a relatively simple construction compared to others in the human frame, it still represents a tremendous engineering challenge to create an adequately functioning artificial equivalent. In total, the design of the new artificial leg and attachments took the pioneering technicians at the Institute of Biotechnology 3 years to complete.

It was 8 years after their initial contact before Brånemark was ready to carry out the surgical procedure on Nilsson. On May 15, 1990, the first stage of surgery was carried out at Carlander's Hospital in Gothenburg, and the skin-penetrating abutment was attached a few months later. On March 7, 1991, Nilsson returned to the hospital for a checkup to ensure that the fixture and the abutment were properly integrated. Within a few weeks the artificial leg was attached. Nilsson had to carry out a careful training regime under the supervision of physiotherapists and the close eye of the engineering technicians. By May 1992, the procedure was completed on her second limb, and she was able to walk on her artificial limbs (Fig 8-4).

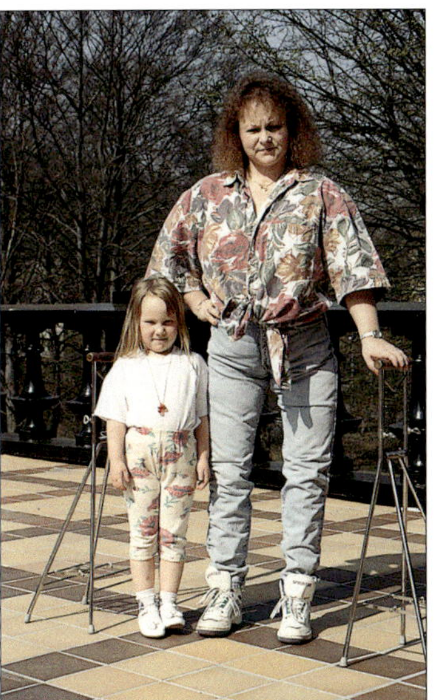

Fig 8-4 Teija Nilsson, with her daughter, standing on her two artificial legs. Without the development of osseointegration to support artificial limbs, she would never have been able to use any type of prosthesis.

Potentially, osseointegrated artificial limbs offer significant benefits when compared to conventional limb designs. The attachment of a lower limb prosthesis, for example, using traditional methods involves pressing the limb stump into a tight-fitting socket. Normally, the stump is covered by a "stump sock" to help prevent the socket rubbing against skin. Then the limb is secured by a complicated system of belts and straps. Frequently, such users still suffer skin soreness and bleeding as the socket rubs against the stumps. The "stump socks" can add to the problem by becoming soaked with sweat and creating additional discomfort, infection, and sometimes an unpleasant smell.

The issue of providing patients with adequate artificial limbs is a controversial one. In the United Kingdom, a report published in March 2000 highlighted serious inadequacies in the provision of help for the disabled in the United Kingdom's hospital system. Basically, it showed that the provision of good quality rehabilitation was a lottery and the luck of geographical location. It revealed wasteful practices, in terms of time and money, that led to many disabled people being provided with ill-fitting and inappropriate aids.

Patients simply will not use artificial limbs if they are not comfortable or fit for the purpose. One young woman explained that she had seven artificial limbs, of which six had been supplied by the National Health System. Only the one she bought privately actually fit and was used regularly. By listening to patients and providing the right equipment and support, money can be saved as well-fitting prostheses obviate the need for repeated hospital visits to sort out problems caused by inadequate rehabilitation.

So far, there have been a limited number of patients provided with lower limb prosthetics based on osseointegration. This is a reflection of Brånemark's natural caution when introducing new clinical applications. These pioneering patients work closely with the medical and support teams so that lessons can be learned and potential problems highlighted. The experience of each new patient is collated and used to improve or modify the technique. Such patients meet annually with the treatment teams. After 10 years of clinical exploration related to osseointegrated retention for limb prostheses, a

development unit called Integrum has been established. Recently, a special unit for orthopedic osseointegration was also organized at Sahlgren's hospital under the leadership of surgeon Rikard Brånemark, Per-Ingvar's son.

Margareta Stenmark is another key patient who has provided important feedback related to osseointegration treatment. When Stenmark was 15, in 1976, she discovered that she had osteosarcoma. She never felt ill but had a little pain and became unsteady on her legs. After experiencing this problem for 3 weeks, she went to the local hospital in Falköping and then to Sahlgren's University Hospital in Gothenburg for a radiograph. Though the doctors did not say anything to her, they told her mother the situation was not so bright. During that time, survival rates for this type of cancer were 20 to 25 percent, but this has since gone up to 60 percent. The incidence of this type of cancer is rare; in Sweden one would expect to see only 15 new children's cases each year.

Stenmark had an operation to remove her affected leg and then underwent chemotherapy. This was a difficult time; she was very tired and lost her hair. She couldn't go out with her friends because of the risk of infection. That said, Stenmark was able to keep "one foot in the world of the living," as she says, because her school friends and teachers made sure she got visits and knew what was going on in school.

During this time, Stenmark also decided she wanted to become a doctor. She jokes that this was some kind of "desire for revenge" on her doctors, but really her ambition was to help other children who might find themselves in a similar situation. She says her revenge lust was more toward the illness than anything else. She has talked about her need to have mental control over her life even when she doesn't have full control over her body. She has fulfilled her ambitions. Stenmark specialized in pediatrics and now works with children with a range of health problems – something she finds quite stimulating.

As a consequence of her disease, Stenmark's leg was amputated quite high up, and she had to learn to walk with a prosthesis. She has talked about the negative aspects of living with a conventional design. "You get a lot of sores on your skin, irritations of the skin, pains in your back, which can make sitting uncomfortable." Her socket also changed shape with the heat or cold. "You can get air in the socket that makes an awful noise. Then there are problems with the ventilation – that cause sweating and unpleasant smells. Because the prosthesis is heavy, you end up walking like a duck," she explains.

In 1990 Stenmark read about Teija Nilsson's operation. Stenmark talked to her doctor and volunteered for the technique. In December 1992, she came for a talk with Brånemark. In February 1993, she had the first operation, followed by the second stage in September 1993. Stenmark explains that one consequence of the operation is that she has had more "phantom pain" in the foot that no longer exists. She got extra physical training to build up the weak muscles.

Stenmark talks about the need for careful hygiene in the area of the implant, and she also uses cream. Being a pioneer, she had to rely on her own knowledge. She believes that there is still much to do when it comes to the external anchorage of the coupling to the titanium. However, Stenmark has noted a number of particular benefits of this type of prosthesis:

1. It is much easier to take on and off. (She always carries the Allen key in her pocket.)
2. The irritating noise has disappeared.
3. No sores.
4. She can walk further without pain.
5. She can bend her knee more easily and fasten her shoes.
6. She can get up and down from the floor more easily (useful when treating children) and does not live in fear that she will lose the prosthesis.
7. She feels some perception and sensation via the prosthesis. She can discriminate between flooring materials, for example.

There have been several other pioneering patients, including a Spanish policeman who on December 23, 1988, stepped on a mine laid by terrorists. He lost the lower part of his leg from the knee. He spent 5 days unconscious, and when he realized he had lost his leg he felt deeply upset. He spent 3 months in the hospital. During the first months he had no problems and healing progressed normally. After about a year he started using a conventional prosthesis. Though the prosthesis functioned well, he says he felt that he couldn't live a normal life. He wanted to be "back to normal." He couldn't wear the prosthesis the whole day because he got pain in his muscles and the skin chafed. He felt tired after wearing it after a while and worried it would come loose.

This patient heard about osseointegration from his dentist. In February 1995 he received the first operation to attach the abutments and has been wearing a new prosthesis since April 1995. He has commented that the osseointegrated prosthesis "feels part of my body." In comparison with the conventional prosthesis he notes, "I have no pain. The only pain is a good pain when I have walked too much. I put this one on at 7 am and take it off at 11 pm. I feel that I know what surface I am stepping on."

Because this prosthesis doesn't have the socket, he does not have the skin problems, the sweat, and the smell. Initially he had a lot of muscle pain and had to get used to a new way of walking. Now he plays table tennis, walks a lot, and swims. He can cycle, but he prefers the motorbike. "I feel more independent now," he says. "I can count on the prosthesis."

Having patients comment with such insight and clarity has resulted in adaptations to the connection mechanism and has also led researchers to look at phenomena such as the ability to perceive sensations that may enhance the use of osseointegration.

Orthopedic applications still face many challenges ahead. This is partly due to the fact that, to be successful, osseointegration requires complete rethinking about connection and loading to provide a secure, long-term method of limb replacement.

Scientific Understanding

Part III

Sense and Sensibility

"If the door of perception were cleansed, everything would appear as it is, infinite."

William Blake, 1757-1827

Osseointegration has shown benefits to patients because it offers a method of providing stable fixation of a variety of prosthetic devices, from a single artificial tooth to a complete artificial leg. Providing a direct replacement for a lost limb or tooth with a restoration of some or all mechanical function is an achievement in itself; however, there appears to be more to osseointegration than simple mechanical issues. There are clear and encouraging signs that osseointegration can provide patients with sensory information, a phenomenon that has been called osseoperception (Fig 9-1).

For researchers working in this clinical field, the key issue is whether or not osseoperception can be exploited positively to create more appropriate prosthetic designs. To do so, we need to understand the mechanisms that support os-seoperception. Researchers worldwide are beginning to study how the body's complex sensory network transmits information and is processed by the brain. This should benefit osseointegration in the long term.

The Beginnings of Osseoperception

In the 1970s, patients started to comment that dental rehabilitation using the osseointegration technique provided them with the feelings and sensations they once had with their own teeth. Many patients commented that they were able to discriminate between the types of food they were eating. Torgny Haraldson was the first to note this in clinical observations. A gifted re-

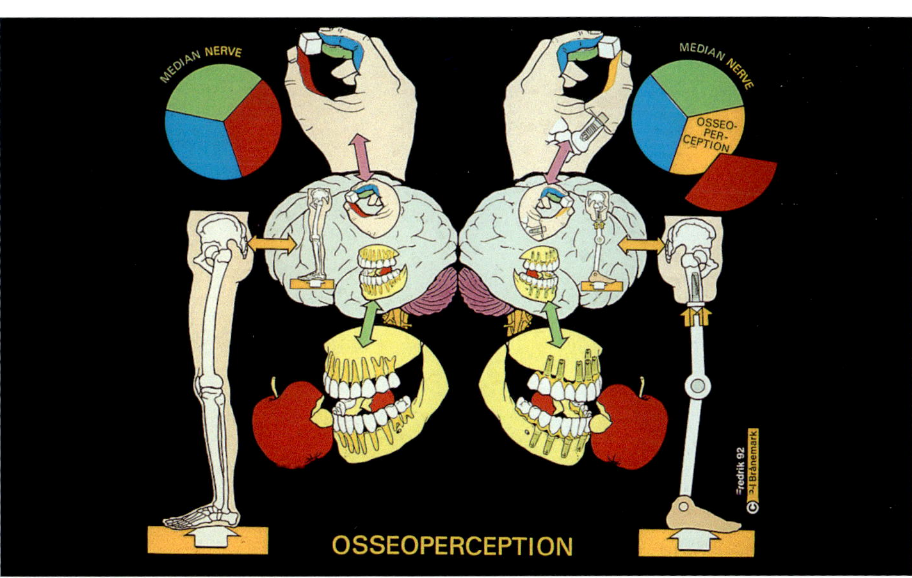

Fig 9-1 Can the flexibility of the brain be exploited to adapt to new situations instead of relying on ingenious engineering devices? Note that osseoperception is a phenomenon that can occur in a number of osseointegration procedures but was first identified in dental applications.

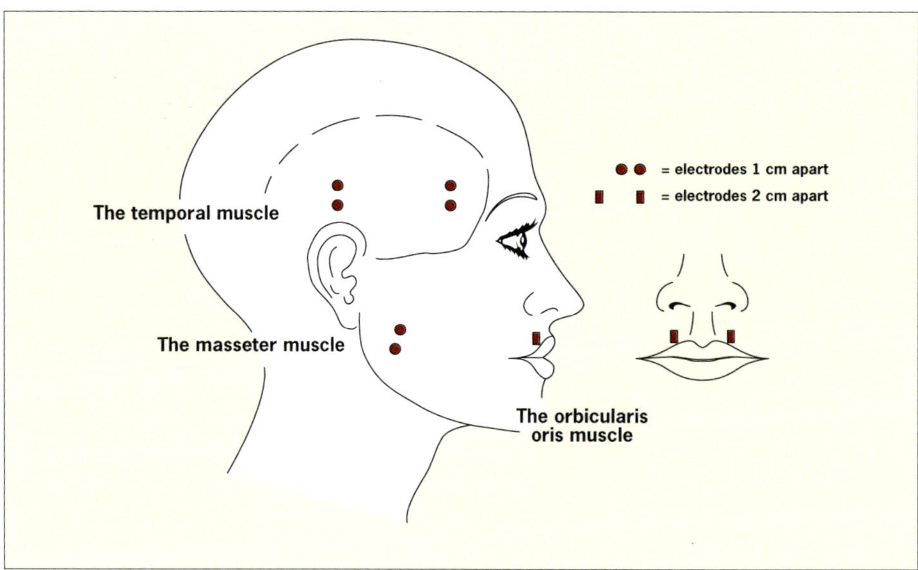

Fig 9-2 By seating electrodes appropriately, Haraldson could measure bite force and compare patients with osseointegrated dental fixtures with those with normal dentition.

searcher and clinician, Haraldson contributed to many areas of research in the dental field. Crucially, his doctoral thesis, completed at Gothenburg University in 1979, was entitled "Functional evaluation of bridges on osseointegrated implants in the edentulous jaw." He found that jawbone-anchored prostheses in the edentulous patient could transmit sensory information, and that these patients achieved a capacity to discriminate the foods they were chewing. This is called osseoperception. It is unclear whether this capacity is an indication of interaction with the nerves or other elements in the jawbone close to, or more distant from, the implanted fixtures (Fig 9-2).

Haraldson established that patients with osseointegrated bridges "have been restored to a level of functional capacity of the masticatory system equal to that in individuals with a natural but reduced dentition of the same extension as in the osseointegration group." Another key observation he noted was that patients with jawbone-anchored bridges and dentate controls have, for all bite force levels tested, equal

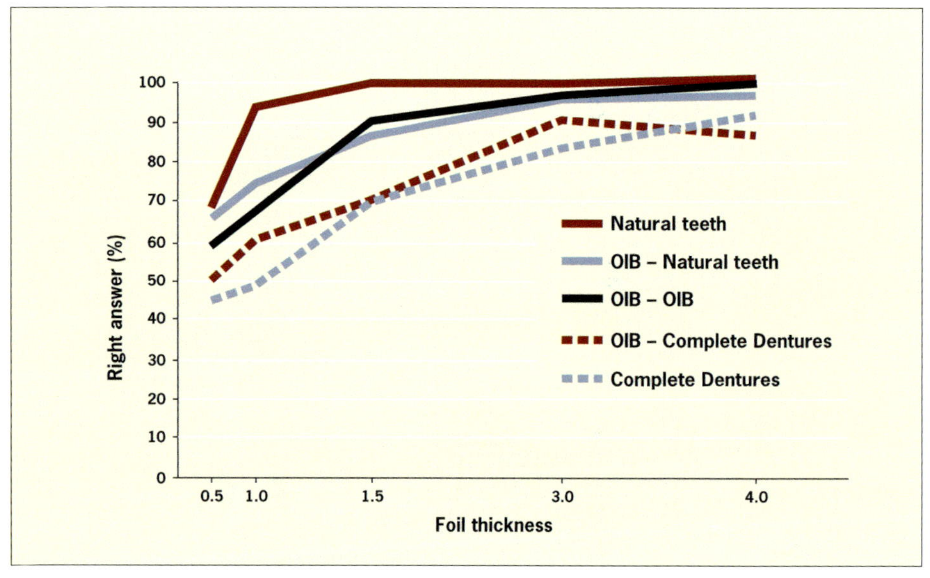

Fig 9-3 Haraldson's work showed the high level of functional capacity gained by patients with osseointegrated dental implants. His work also noted a phenomenon that has now been dubbed osseoperception. (OIB) Osseointegrated bone.

bite force capacity, in some cases as high as a maximal bite force capacity in young, healthy individuals. Further he noted, "Patients with jawbone-anchored bridges had the same ability to discriminate between bite force levels and showed a reflex activity with the same characteristics as dentate controls with the same extension of the dentition" (Fig 9-3).

For dental patients, the notion of osseoperception has raised many questions. Researchers wonder what happens in the cortical area of the brain when teeth are lost, what is the capacity to retain control and function, how does the sensory region of the brain deal with reduced dentition, and can training or rehabilitation overcome lost control and function. Then there is the question of whether or not osseoperception can be used for the benefit of the patient. Currently, researchers have become interested in osseoperception because they are exploring the possibility of whether or not the phenomenon can be exploited to improve the function of the prosthetic design. Researchers are now considering whether there is a correlation between the kind of sensory rehabilitation for dental patients that has been demonstrated by Haraldson and the sensory experiences noted in limb amputees with osseointegrated prosthetics. If that is the case, this may open up tremendous opportunities for all types of amputees, not only dental patients.

Beyond Dentistry

Similar ability to demonstrate a sensory capacity via an osseointegrated prosthesis has been shown in other types of patients. Limb amputee patients have also commented on an increased ability to "feel" with an osseointegrated prosthesis. One patient with an above-knee amputation fitted with an osseointegrated prosthesis pointed out, "I can now feel what kind of surface my prosthetic foot touches" (Figs 9-4a and 9-4b). Another patient claimed to feel the sensation of raindrops falling on his prosthetic foot.

In lower-limb amputees, this could mean the development of artificial limbs offering improved gait, and for upper-limb patients, better control of arms and hands. Just how to exploit osseoperception in this context is still uncertain. Whatever benefits are to be gained must be considered with the overall improvements to be achieved by using the osseointegration technique as an anchorage point for a prosthesis.

Researchers say there are a number of hypothetical advantages of an osseointegrated amputation prosthesis. These include:

- A direct transfer of load to the skeleton
- Little or no risk of mechanical skin irritation or nerve compression by the prosthesis socket
- Eliminated need for prosthetic exchange due to stump shape or configuration alterations
- Optimum control of prosthetic movement because of the stable fixation to the skeleton of the stump
- Restoration of some sensory and tactile function, (osseoperception)

For limb amputees, vibrometric analysis has been one of the methods used to evaluate osseoperception. The technique is based on methods developed by Göran Lundborg in 1986 and

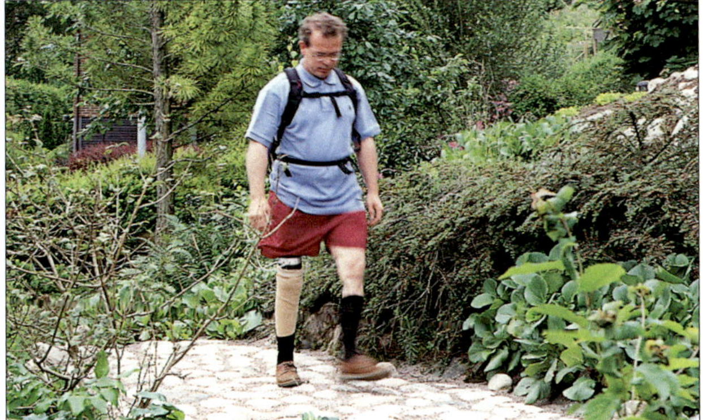
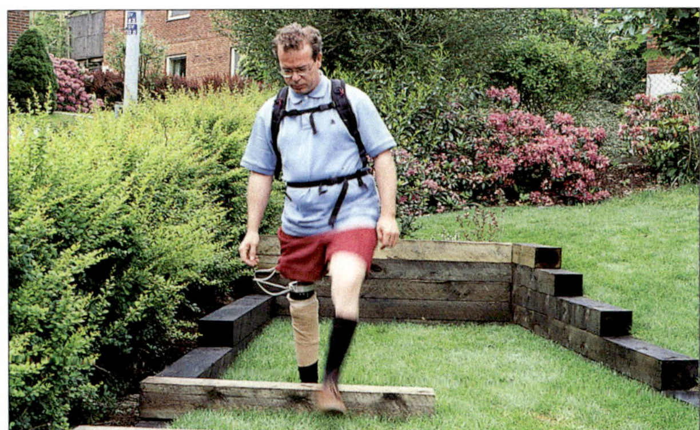

Figs 9-4a and **9-4b** The ability to discriminate between different surfaces is part of the osseoperception experience.

was originally used to evaluate sensory function in relation to compression neuropathy such as carpal tunnel syndrome. It has been modified for use with prosthetic hands.

The technique employs a small device with a vibrating tip that can deliver a range of frequencies from 8 to 250 Hz to the prosthetic components or directly to the abutment. This helps evaluate the capacity of the hand and demonstrate the patient's ability to feel stimuli applied to either the extremity or the prosthetic device itself. The results showed the perception of vibration in the hand of an osseointegrated prosthesis corresponded to that of a normal hand, while in patients wearing a conventional prosthesis the perception of vibration was reduced to 70 percent of that of a normal hand. When the vibrations were applied directly to the osseointegrated fixture, rather than the prosthesis, the vibration was felt more strongly than either the normal hand or the prosthesis. These results indicate that bone tissue appears to have the ability, if properly loaded, to detect and transfer vibratory stimuli to the nervous system.

Issues for Future Study

Based on these results, researchers say that osseoperception is a clinical reality. The underlying mechanisms, however, have yet to be identified. Researchers, such as Professor Björn Rydevik in Gothenburg, point out that there might be proprioceptive inputs from muscle spindle receptors and mechanoreceptors in the joint that are activated by the direct loading onto bone tissue. To establish clear mechanisms, researchers believe they need to look closely at mechanoreceptors in bone and neurons containing neuropeptides. Currently, researchers do not understand the relative roles of these in relation to the periosteum and the skin. The interactions between the osseointegrated fixture, bone tissue, various receptor systems, and the peripheral and central nervous system are clearly of interest in this context.

Today, researchers believe that by studying sensory pathways and learning more about the basic systems that transmit such information to the brain, they can gain clues about the mechanisms that support osseoperception. For example, Professor Robert Myers, of the department of anesthesiology and neuropathology at the Virginia Medical Center and the University of California, La Jolla, is studying the osseoperception phenomenon from the context of pain. His group has developed successful models of neuropathic pain in rodents over the last decade. The group believes that this has given new understanding about the relationship between peripheral immune events, neural remodeling, and perception. The goal is to continue this research to find out how injured bone or remodeled bone may change the anatomical structure and sensory pathways serving perception.

One way to do this is to look at other anatomical structures. Our skin has many types of receptors. Pacini and Meissener receptors pick up pressure and touch, while Merkel and Ruffini receptors respond to constant loading. Currently, no one is entirely sure how they correspond to receptors in the bone and marrow. This is an obvious area for further study.

Of course, any discussion about osseoperception must consider the role of the brain in interpreting sensory information and the pathways that transmit such information. We know that the brain, through the somatosensory brain cortex, has dedicated maps that help in the interpretation of sensory messages from different parts of the body (Fig 9-5). Humans already have sophisticated sensory mechanisms that combine physical detection with interpretation from the brain. The brain has a tremendous capacity, a plasticity, to adapt to changed circumstances and to alter its own map of the body to refine its control mechanisms.

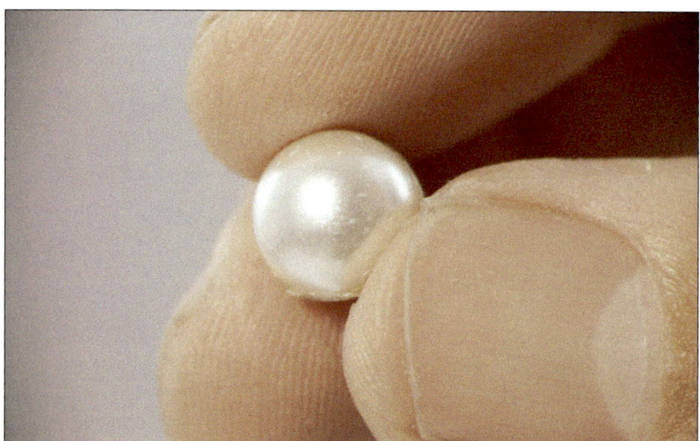

Fig 9-5 The sense of touch requires an interaction between the hand and the brain. Tactile receptors are located in the fingertips, but the inner picture of an object is located in the brain and has been learned by experience.

Naturally, the hands are allocated a large area of the cortex to accommodate the huge amount of data they produce. While vision can register a wealth of information about the world around us, and experience of previous encounters with objects provides us with expectations, our hands provide us with detailed information about the true nature of objects. The seemingly simple action of holding an object can reveal most of its secrets — weight, density, texture, and viscosity — that cannot be discovered by sight alone. The subtlety and sophistication of this ability is still not entirely understood. Neither is proprioception — the ability to gauge position and movement. Today we are starting to learn how proprioception is achieved. For a long time proprioception was believed to be based on receptors in joint capsules, periarticular structures, tendons, and muscles. More recent research has shown that proprioception is mainly based on Ruffini receptors in the skin responding to tension and stretching forces (Fig 9-6).

In regard to osseoperception, Brånemark himself has also noted the difficulties. On September 16, 1998, he noted, "Owing to the nature of osseointegration, it is not easy to dissect the system of anchorage from the clinical level down to the molecular level or even the real interface, which is still largely a mystery." Björn Rydevik has noted in his work that "the interactions between the osseointegrated fixtures, the bone tissue, the various receptor systems, and the peripheral and

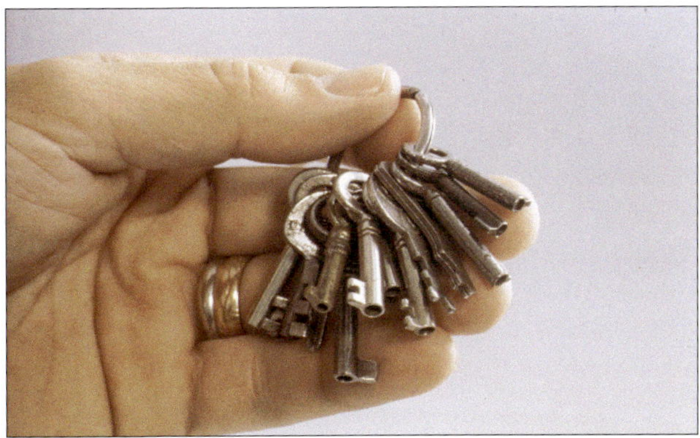

Fig 9-6 Sensory stimuli, together with memory programs, are important factors in the ability to feel and identify objects, such as picking a single key out of several.

central nervous systems, constitute critical factors in this regard." Brånemark and his colleagues worldwide feel that osseoperception, once understood, can be employed to the benefit of patients. They regard osseoperception as important for amputees as it provides a level of function that appears not to be possible with conventional prosthetic solutions.

For the patients themselves, there are tremendous emotional benefits to be gained. The sensations they feel through, by, or with their various prostheses are an affirmation that their implanted components have been accepted by their own tissues and are now an integral part of their bodies. This enhances their sense of well-being and self-esteem, which is not to be underestimated as part of the overall treatment outcome.

10 The Biomechanical Approach

"It is a capital mistake to theorize before one has data."

Sir Arthur Conan Doyle, 1859-1930

The success of osseointegration in clinical application is as much due to the mechanical design of the components as it is to the gentle surgical techniques that have evolved. Per-Ingvar Brånemark knew osseointegration required a multidisciplinary approach, and he recruited world-class researchers in other fields to help him understand all aspects of the work.

This has been a highly effective strategy. Early work, led by Richard Skalak in the late 1960s, identified the mechanical characteristics of implant designs and noted the strength of such devices once successfully integrated into healthy bone (Fig 10-1). Today, of course, we have 30 years of experience with patients who have osseointegrated fixtures in their jaws to support this work.

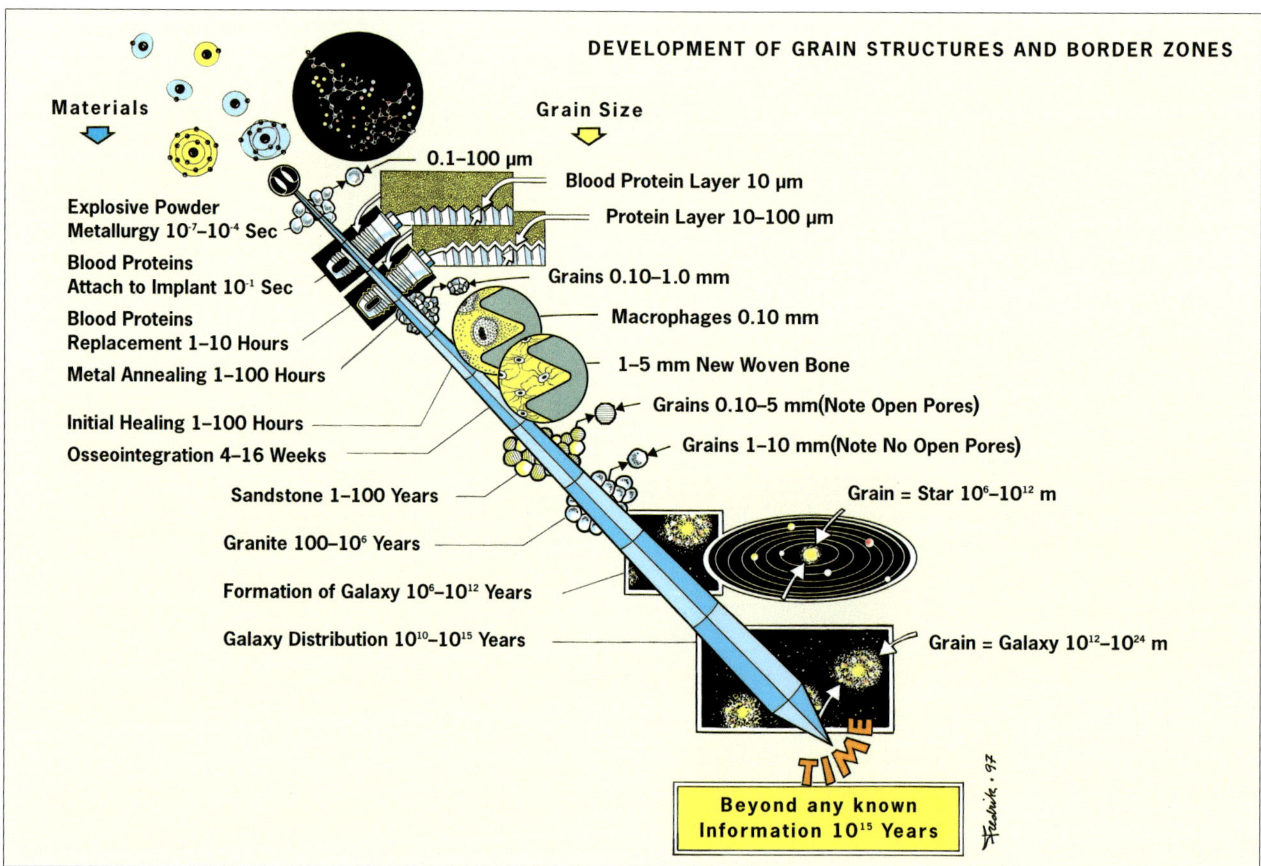

Fig 10-1 Richard Skalak attempted to stimulate thought among the scientific community by comparing processes involved in osseointegration with other processes that occur at different scales.

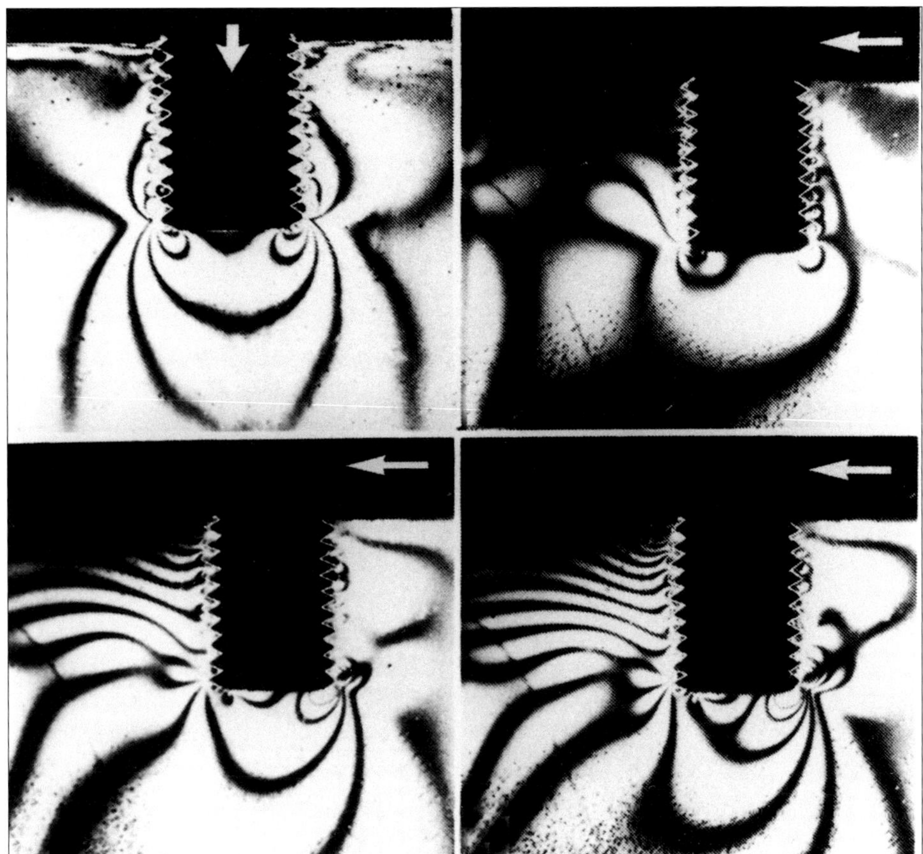

Fig 10-2 Haraldson's study of the stresses surrounding test implants at different loads. Note the difference in the fringe pattern between the axial and horizontal loads.

By the early 1990s, the study of the biomechanics of osseointegration had entered a new phase. In 1994, Richard Skalak noted, "In the early phase of clinical experience with osseointegrated prostheses, the emphasis was on questions of initial stability." This was then accompanied by "achieving a functional osseointegration in the first few weeks after placement of screws or other fixation devices." Now the emphasis has shifted to the long-term performance, and remodeling, of bone after osseointegration has been achieved.

As dental rehabilitation was the first clinical application of osseointegration, scientists have gained a considerable amount of information about its biomechanical behavior in this regard. The distribution of bite forces by a dental prosthesis to each of the supporting fixtures has been examined in detail by theoretic studies and proven by successful clinical application to be capable of providing a reliable functional load transfer without progressive damage or loosening. Torgny Haraldson carried out a study of biomechanics of oral implants of various designs in the 1970s. His work showed that pretapping and careful insertion of a threaded implant could reduce stresses in the surrounding test piece. These results had important clinical relevance (Fig 10-2).

The implications of modifications to the implant surface such as roughness, porosity, and coatings have been studied. So far, the evidence is not clear whether such modifications have any major advantages over machined titanium surfaces. Skalak carried out many studies of the titanium surface with a scanning electron microscope, for example, which supports the notion that the original surface developed for the fixtures functions well. Specifically, Skalak and a co-worker, Y. Zhao, produced two papers relating to surface characteristics. One was entitled "Interaction of Force-Fitting and Surface Roughness of Implants" and the other was "Similarity in Stress Distribution in Bone for Various Implant Surface Roughness Heights of Similar Form." Both papers were published in 2000.

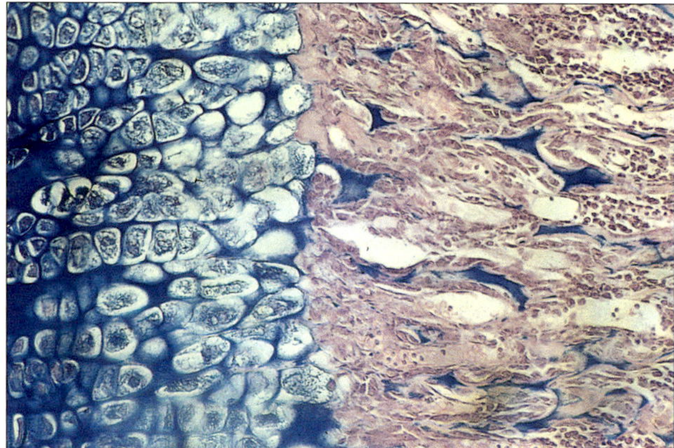

Fig 10-3   Normal bone growth.

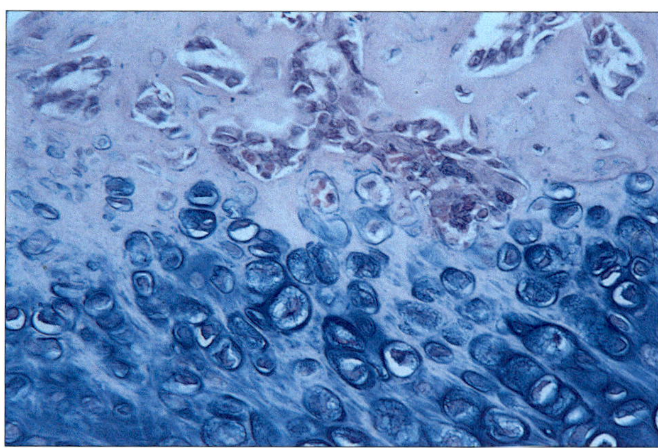

Fig 10-4   Endochondral bone formation following a fracture.

Direct bone attachment can be successful under a variety of conditions. In 1994, Skalak noted that "satisfactory initial stability and a subsequent firm osseointegration has been demonstrated in hand surgery, in ankle joint replacement, and in amputees in both upper and lower limbs." Skalak felt that, with careful installation of fixtures and a period of several weeks with either zero or moderate loads, osseointegration could be achieved in most bones of the human frame.

That said, the success of implants in other regions of the body has been mixed both for traditional joint and limb replacement and for osseointegration. Brånemark and Skalak have realized that understanding why some implants fail in some patients holds important lessons for the improvement in osseointegration outside the dental field. Of most interest to researchers are issues of long-term prognosis and implant design in relation to failure phenomena. Such failures include atrophy or resorption of bone because of stress shielding. There are other long-term effects such as fatigue, corrosion failure, and inflammation and loosening due to product wear.

Osseointegration or Pseudoarthrosis

The basic requirements for successful osseointegration are well understood. One important factor is careful surgery that uses low drilling speeds and temperature controls to minimize trauma to the remaining bone. Initial mechanical stability is also important. The shapes of the titanium screws are designed to provide a high pull-out strength.

In dental applications, experience has shown that after the insertion of a fixture, osseointegration was successful provided there was a period of no loading or very light loading. If loading was excessive at the early stages of an implant being installed, osseointegration was not achieved. Instead, a fibrous capsule formed around the implant. Though this phenomenon is well known, researchers do not yet have the quantitative data to help clinicians predict either the timing or loading levels that can guarantee osseointegration.

The underlying cause for the production of fibrous tissue or bone has been a matter of conjecture. One possible explanation for the production of fibrous tissue at an implant surface is that it is sensitive to the micromotion of the implant relative to the surrounding bone. In fracture healing, for example, it has been suggested that the creation of bone or fibrous tissue is similar to that of the processes of tissue differentiation during embryonic development. Bone will be produced if the shear and hydrostatic stresses are within certain limits, while the influence of larger cyclical stresses results in the production of fibrous tissue or cartilage, depending on the degree of vascularity. Failing integration in bone, to some extent, resembles failed healing of a fracture that leads to pseudoarthrosis (Figs 10-3 and 10-4).

Effects of Stress and Fatigue

In some joint replacement applications, such as hip and knee, there is also the problem of mechanical wear to be considered. Generally, the effects of wear are mainly inflammation and immunologic responses. The production of wear products tends to be mechanical in nature and, as such, does not directly involve the mechanics of the bone or the interface between the implant and bone.

Some progress has been made in understanding stress shielding and fatigue in relation to osseointegration. The bulk of the knowledge comes from the dental experience. It has been found that stress shielding and fatigue are not necessarily limiting factors for the successful function of a dental prosthesis. Stress shielding has been found to reduce bone height around individual dental fixtures. This does not appear to be progressive in nature and seems to stabilize at 1 or 2 mm after a period of about a year. Studies have been trying to establish whether or not this bone loss is due to stress shielding or to so-called microdamage caused by overstressing the bone. As the range of applications for osseointegration grows, learning more about factors such as stress shielding and related problems that can lead to long-term resorption is becoming even more important (Fig 10-5).

Bone response to stress is essentially of two types – internal remodeling and surface remodeling. Internal remodeling normally refers to a change of density, porosity, or rearrangement of internal geometry such as trabeculae. Surface remodeling involves the removal or addition of bone to the periosteal surface so that the cross section of the bone is altered.

Wolff's Law

There are some basic concepts about bone loading that form the foundation for current work. Wolff's Law is one of the early known works on bone loading and was first postulated in 1892. This states that bone remodels in response to the stress applied to it. As we know, bone is in a constant state of repair, renewal, and remodeling according to the demands placed on it. Though Wolff's Law is a hypothesis that is generally accepted, it has not been possible to establish any particular factor controlling the adaptation of bone to mechanical load. Researchers recognize that such adaptation is a key factor for the long-term success of osseointegration, particularly in orthopedic applications.

It is clear that life-long remodeling of the skeleton affects implanted devices. Researchers have gained a better understanding about remodeling processes and measure its effect through bone-mineral determinations. How mechanical stimuli interact with the mechanical response is being studied. Findings from the mid-1990s indicate that clinicians may be able to adapt the remodeling process by exposing bones to repetitive strains of different frequencies. Repetitive loading of the skeleton has the effect of causing both macro- and micro fatigue fractures.

We can learn much from materials technology and the behavior of non-biological materials. Most metals and plastic suffer fatigue when subjected to repeated stress at lower levels. The peak stress required to cause fatigue failure decreases with the number of cycles of loading. It can be a fraction of the original stress values when thousands or even millions of cycles have been completed. In inert materials, fatigue failure begins with the formation of microcracks within the material or on its surface. The cracks progressively enlarge, leading to subsequent failure. Fatigue failure does pose a clinically significant problem as it occurs in metal, ceramic, and bone cement.

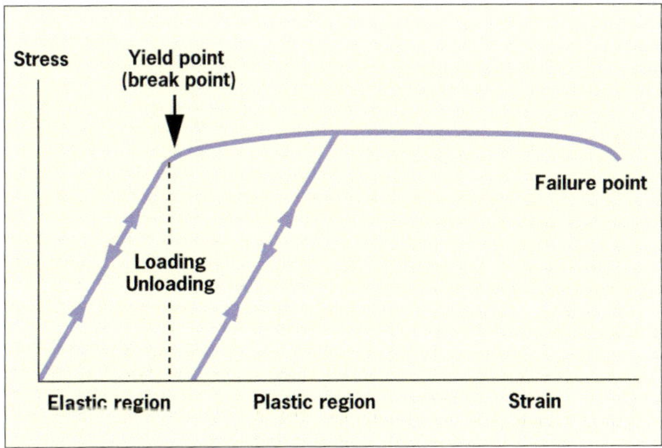

Fig 10-5 The mechanical properties of bone can be described by the same variables as any other material.

Mechanics of Bone Remodeling

A load on skeletal tissue will deform or strain the tissue. This stretches the loaded tissue, which resists with an elastic force called stress. Researchers have found that strain, rather than stress, appears to control and generate the stimuli that control biological reactions as a result of mechanical loads. It seems that biological tissue aims at creating an optimized shape and structure for bone that once achieved helps minimize the impact of strain and ensure the correct amount of bone mineral.

Bone remodeling is a very adaptive process though with a short memory. This means that activity and correct loading are necessary for a human to maintain bone density. Use it or lose it.

Some researchers say that remodeling takes place through the basic metabolic units. This is an orderly sequence of events beginning with activation-resorption-formation. Here, activation involves the triggering of the resorptive ability of the basic metabolic unit. Resorption results in cavities when part of the bone matrix is removed. This resorptive or osteoclastic activity is coupled with the subsequent formative or osteoblastic activity (Fig 10-6). The final result of this activation-resorption-formation sequence is a basic metabolic unit. It has been estimated that the skeleton of a normal adult will create many millions of basic metabolic units each year. The activation-resorption-formation cycle takes about 4 months.

Living bone and inert, biological materials clearly differ in that bone has the inherent capacity of self-repair and regeneration. In this regard, a homeostatic state is possible for bone, where the rate of stress-related damage is balanced by the rate of bone repair. Recently researchers have begun to believe that the flow of fluid in the tiny channels within bone (the canaliculi), which connect to the lacunae where the cell is located, might be one possible signal mechanism for the bone to adjust and remodel in an adequate manner (Figs 10-7 and 10-8).

Researchers need to learn the conditions needed to create optimized, stable bone. They want to establish the details of the ways in which stress and strain are sensed by bone and the metabolic pathways that allow remodeling to take place.

A fascinating aspect of bone remodeling is the role of sensors and responding elements. It is believed that osteocytes, for example, as they are regularly distributed and interconnected, may be the mechanoreceptors in bone. This interconnection allows the osteocytes to respond to stresses applied over some finite area rather than to the stress at the cell body only.

Researchers believe that bone remodeling by osteoblasts and osteoclasts will have some limited region of response rather than only at one point. It has been established that the range of sensing and response has been useful in the simulation of bone remodeling. In relation to this, Richard Skalak wrote, "In morphology, it is shown that the size and branching of trabeculae depends on the spacing of the mechanotransducers and the range of influence of the repairing elements. In view of the complexities of the bone responses and the paucity of detailed knowledge of these processes, prediction of long-term outcomes of particular cases and new prosthetic designs is not yet possible with reliable accuracy."

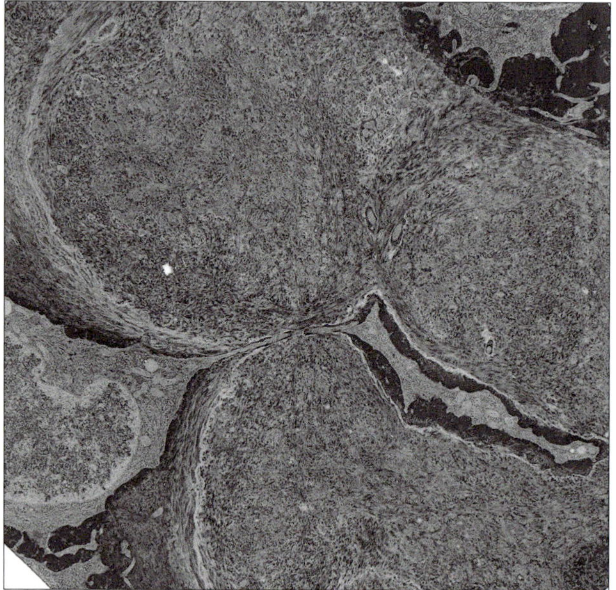

Fig 10-6   Canaliculi lying within the bone structure.

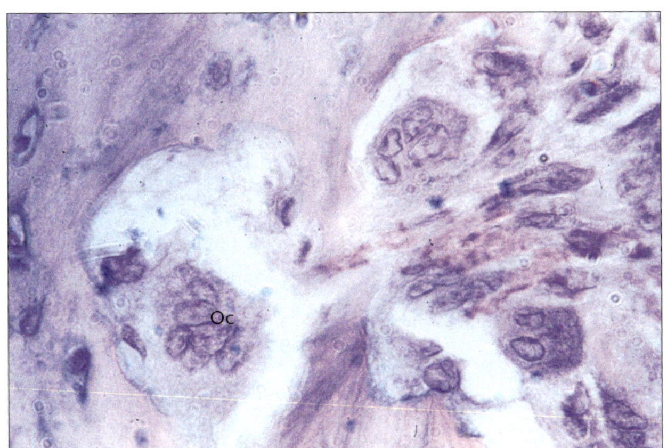

Fig 10-7 An osteoclast (Oc) cell lies close to Howship's lacuna while an osteoblast can be seen within the bone matrix.

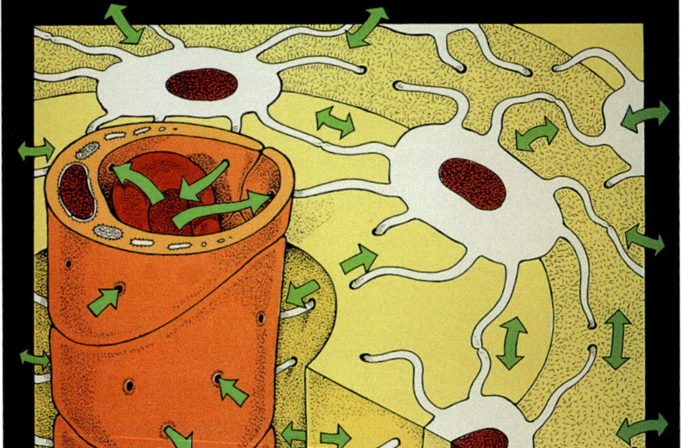

Fig 10-8 The fluid flow in the canaliculi, which interconnect the osteocytes with the central vascular canal, generates a shear stress, which is believed to be a primary stimulus for bone remodeling.

Research Discoveries

There is a close relationship between strain history and the way in which bone adjusts its structure and mineral content. Researchers still admit that the mechanisms that transfer mechanical events into biologic responses at the bone cell level remain unresolved. It has been found that bone is sensitive to mechanical strains up to at least 60 Hz and that high frequency strains (15 to 50 Hz) happen in the human skeleton during normal activities. Further bone sensitivity to mechanical strain is frequency dependent.

Researchers have been developing methods to assess bone mineral content and factors that influence it. New tools have become available such as the absorptimetric technique that allows bone remodeling to be observed in humans and other mammals. Biochemical markers can also be used to study bone remodeling. Such markers include substances that are released during bone resorption and formation. Different molecules can be used as markers to identify the various aspects of bone turnover. Some are by-products formed during resorption or formation, while others reflect enzymatic activities in bone cells.

When it comes to stress, design of the prosthesis is a key issue. A subtle balance in the transfer of functional load to the interface between fixture and bone is crucial so there is neither over- nor underload. In many prosthetic designs that have a connection directly to bone, some regions of the bone may not experience normal stress levels. Too little or too much load can both have adverse results. In regions of low stress, bone may atrophy, which is clinically identified as bone loss. Normally this can be observed in the proximal region of the implant. Again, though the basic supposition is generally accepted to be a clinical reality, a detailed quantitative evaluation has yet to lead to predictive formulae. Once this has been achieved, it may be possible to use such a tool systemically for the detailed design and development of orthopedic implants such that long-term bone resorption can be accurately predicted and controlled.

Some simplified models of hip prostheses, for example, have indicated what the stress distribution in bone is like. However, while such models serve to illustrate the basic phenomena of stress shielding, the reality is far more complex. More detailed analyses are required before implant designs can be based directly on theoretical analyses.

A technique used for analyzing engineering structures, called finite element analysis, is being applied to study stress distribution and subsequent bone remodeling. As for any theoretical modeling, some assumptions or criteria have to be made if a realistic model for bone resorption caused by stress shielding is to be achieved. The location and shape of the bone and the activity being carried out will mean that any forces applied will vary in magnitude, duration, and direction. Even today researchers are not entirely sure which loading characteristics are key to bone remodeling.

With these issues in mind, computational analysis techniques can provide three-dimensional models that accurately reflect stress distribution of a particular implant and bone geometry.

Certain assumptions are made relating to bone remodeling behavior in response to stress. Generally it is assumed that bones will not atrophy or augment if the stress applied to a bone is within some normal range. Lower stress levels may cause bone to atrophy and, for higher stresses than normal, bone may augment. For bone atrophy or growth, stress distribution alters and may cause further changes of form or density. These changes can be charted iteratively by computer simulations. Such cycles are repeated until either failure occurs or a steady state is achieved.

Still to Be Revealed

Currently research has not revealed any deep understanding of what happens when stress is applied to a specific point in bone or the influence of different patterns of stress as a function of time. This lack of knowledge is being addressed. It is important because cycles of different stress patterns may have an influence on the overall success of osseointegration.

Researchers are fine-tuning their computational methods and comparing them against experimental data. The parameters used in analysis techniques need to be adjusted to take into account different types of bone, age, and other conditions.

The current level of knowledge relating to computer analysis techniques and materials technology is sufficient for the design of prosthetic elements of suitable strength and fatigue life under prescribed loading conditions and a degree of osseointegration. Coupled with experience in surgical techniques and the behavior of biomaterials, this can ensure osseointegration in any appropriate skeletal component. Stress distributions in bone for complete osseointegration can be reliably calculated. The limits, however, of the stress and strain that may be applied without hindering the development of osseointegration are not entirely established.

Studies have established that bone loss caused by stress shielding observed clinically may be reproduced theoretically by making the assumption that understressed regions of a bone will be resorbed by the body over time. Quantifying resorption is still beyond current knowledge as it relies on several parameters of sensing and response processes. These processes have not been established with sufficient accuracy to predict resorption in individual patients, although general trends can be established. Such trends are useful when considering prosthetic designs.

The way to improve prosthetics for individual needs is to look further into the processes behind transduction and bone growth.

11

At the Cellular Level

"The truth is rarely pure, and never simple."

Oscar Wilde, 1854-1900

For the past decade or so, increased efforts have been directed toward understanding the molecular and cellular processes that support osseointegration. Despite nearly 4 decades of clinical experience, this continues to be a major gap in the knowledge where there are more questions than answers.

Richard Skalak, in a personal letter to the author on December 8, 1996, pointed out that "a detailed understanding of molecular and cellular events is necessary for further rational improvements and procedures." He supported Per-Ingvar Brånemark's desire to seek scientists in such fields to examine this aspect of osseointegration. As a start, the Institute for Applied Biotechnology in Sweden, in collaboration with the Institute for Mechanics and Materials at the University of California, San Diego, held a small workshop on the topic in London on September 22-23, 1995.

Brånemark hopes that better knowledge of the basic mechanisms will lead to a reduction in the healing period after osseointegrative procedures and a simplification of the total construction of implants. Some of the issues Brånemark and his colleagues are seeking to address include discovering the critical conditions for close apposition of regenerated bone at the interface of the implants and the absence of any intermediate soft tissue or fibrous layer at the interface. In osseointegration procedures, over time, there is no continuous marginal destruction of bone. This is an important factor in the success of the technique as a whole, but the reason for it has not been identified (Fig 11-1).

When it comes to soft tissue, there are also a number of issues to be studied. This includes discovering why soft tissue does not recognize the implant as a foreign body and why the epithelium does not grow down around a titanium implant as it does with other implanted materials.

The researchers are eager to understand other aspects such as the response of bone and soft tissue after irradiation, rheumatoid arthritis, or osteoporosis. At the clinical level, it has been demonstrated that irradiated bone close to the rheumatoid sites can still develop a firm and useful osseointegration, but we do not know what the cell responses are in these situations.

Whenever a fixture is inserted into bone there is always some damage to the supporting bone tissue. Following this there is repair, remodeling, and regeneration controlled by a variety of mechanisms. Growth factors and genetic responses to the epigenetic factors regulate developments. So far, however, the details of signal transduction, molecular messengers, and cellular responses *in vivo* are not really understood. The goal of current research is to focus on the cellular and molecular levels of the target tissues at the implant site with the ultimate aim of controlling more effectively those cellular activities that influence osseointegration.

Researchers are eager to understand tissue function for a number of reasons, not simply to facilitate osseointegration but to intervene in a variety of diseases. Molecular probes of different types allow the nature of tissue function to be explored. Cell mapping techniques are also beginning to help us learn about the details of the cell, the close territorial matrix, and the distant interterritorial matrix. Researchers are now able to identify the differences in the organization and cellular components at these different sites and detail their structure.

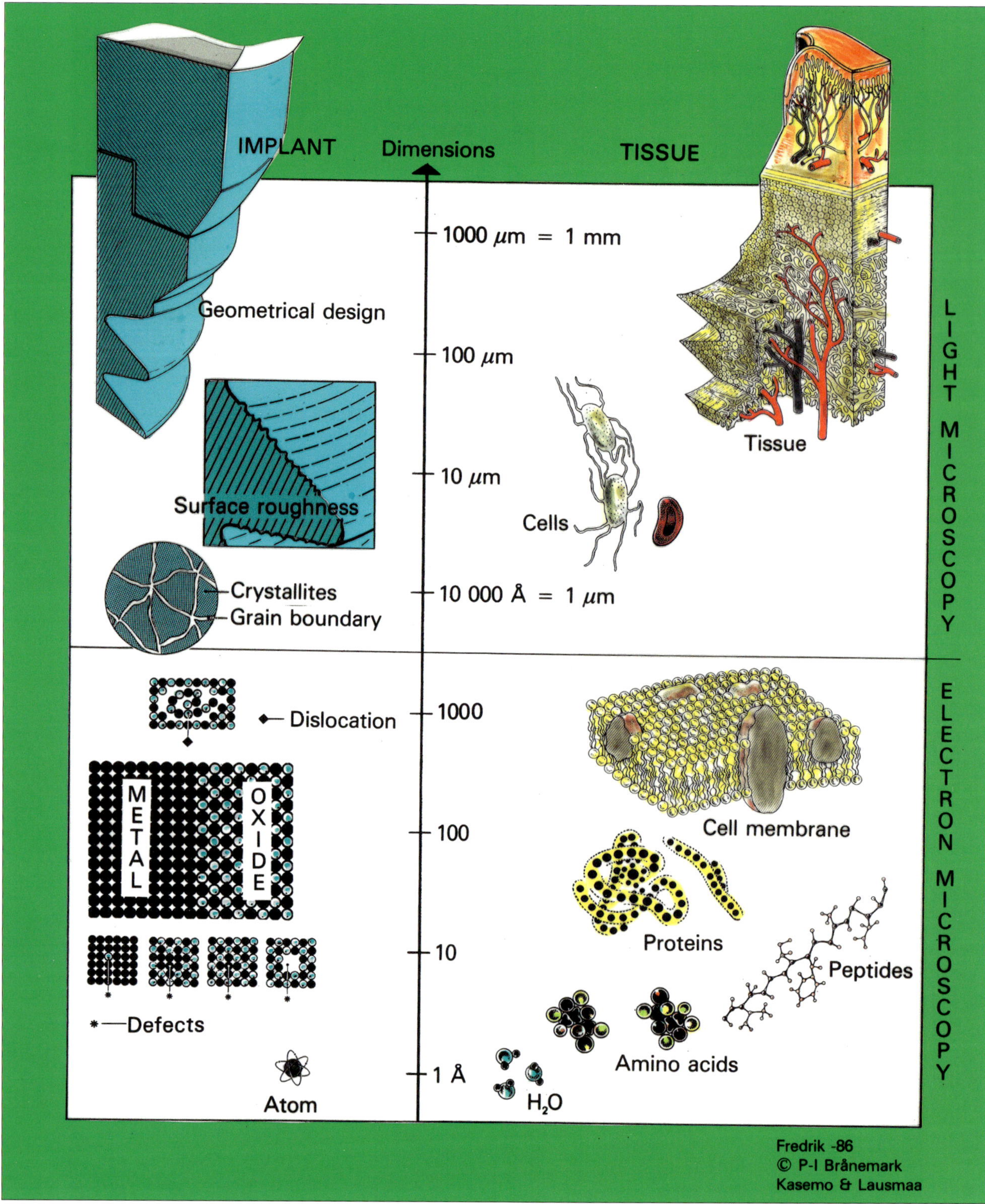

Fig 11-1   Produced in 1986, this is a schematic illustration of some relevant structures of the biomaterial-biosystem interface and their approximate linear dimensions.

Tissue Structure

Generally all types of tissue have similar and related building blocks. These are the molecular constituents. Unlike the uniformity of an implant component, tissues are not homogeneous. This may, one day, be a consideration in future implant material design. Connective tissue, for example, is the most abundant and widely distributed type of tissue in the body. It is present in skin, membranes, muscles, bone, and nerves, as well as all internal organs. This type of tissues exists as delicate webs that can hold together internal organs and give them their shape. In other parts of the body, connective tissue is in the form of tough ropes, rigid bones, and even exists as a fluid – blood, a mobile tissue.

The job of connective tissue is as diverse as its appearance. It connects other tissues together and forms a supporting framework for the entire body and for individual organs. As blood, it provides a means to transport substances throughout the body. Connective tissue, like most tissues, is made up of a variety of cells within an intercellular material called matrix. In addition, most tissues contain fibers and large anionic proteoglycans that contribute negative fixed charges for the regulation of water retention, sugars, and flux.

Tissues such as cartilage, for example, show a difference in cell populations as you look from the superficial to the deeper layers of the tissue. Within the cell matrix, further differences are created by variation in molecular constituents according to their position relative to their cells. These molecules, however, are made by the cells to create a tissue. Looking at the example of cartilage, cells assemble the collagen fibers that are covered by molecules to form a network. Collagen fibers have different dimensions according to their location, a feature that is tightly regulated by the cell itself. The properties of the tissue depend on the overall matrix. By monitoring events at the cell surface, including biomechanical aspects, information is revealed about what is happening within the cell.

Response to Implants

The cell's response to implants varies according to the nature of the ligand in the matrix. Upon binding, one of two pathways is activated. One pathway heads toward the cytoskeleton and leads to growth, migration, and/or cell division. The other pathway is believed to induce the production of saccharides and proteins to repair or break down the surrounding matrix. Adrian Parsegian proposed this idea at a symposium in London in 1995.

Over the years, a certain amount of information about the interface between the titanium implant component and the adjacent tissue has been learned. One of the keys to successful osseointegration has been in the selection and surface preparation of the material used. Pure titanium has proved to be most successful in this respect. In open air, pure titanium will rapidly develop a thin oxide layer, which then grows slowly over time. When a fixture is inserted in bone and tissue it presents a surface more akin to ceramic than metal.

Titanium behaves differently in the human body than in air. In addition to forming a titanium peroxide gel layer in the body, titanium also diffuses into surrounding tissue. When a titanium implant is installed, the body's defense mechanism is activated and produces free oxygen radicals that speed up the oxidation of the metal. Usually, when the titanium component is inserted, the oxide layer is approximately 20 atoms thick. In a relatively short period of time, this layer increases to the depth of about 500 atoms. What appears to happen is that during this oxidation, and in the presence of these free radicals, the titanium combines to form a number of titanium peroxide complexes. It has been suggested that a titanium peroxide gel may form at the surface of the titanium oxide. Hydrogen peroxide may be the cause of the thicker layer *in vivo*, particularly where an implant may be in contact with marrow. The gel produced may be mitigating the effects of nitric oxide production by the reparative cells. This appears to cut off the inflammation processes around the site of the implant and help promote healing.

Also, the way in which the titanium surface is cleaned before insertion makes a difference in what happens initially. Complement factor is deposited first and replaced by fibrinogen after about 1 minute through a phenomenon called the Vroman effect. Antibodies to these molecules are found in later stages. In principle, it should be possible to discover the sequences of proteins and antibodies that are formed, although the task is complex because several species are involved and it is difficult to identify a single layer and complexes acting as a unit. Cells, which begin to adhere within about 30 seconds, have multiple attachment points, and there is an optimal packing of receptor molecules on the implant surface for cell adhesion. Researchers want to know whether other materials initiate the same response, and if they don't, then what is unique about titanium. As has been noted, surface treatment can also play a role in influencing initial events, so further studies are aimed at comparing different types of surface treatments as well as other kinds of metals.

Researchers believe that the molecular behavior of proteins, particularly glycoproteins, and some saccharides adhering to titanium oxide are key in determining early implant success. We still have little idea about the initial events that take place, apart from the fact that proteins are involved and that a conditioning film of glycoproteins generally forms first. Further research may seek to establish the message channel by which information from this film is broadcast to the level of the cells through this conditioning film.

Another aspect of osseointegration is that of bioadhesion, which tends not to be linear with regard to surface energy. In an osteosarcoma cell, there is always a film 100 to 200 angstrom thick between the cell and a surface to which it adheres. *In vivo*, many proteins from the bone and blood may be involved in creating such a layer. Bioadhesion takes place in a dry microenvironment, and water has to be totally removed from the system or there will be no interaction between cells. Even a layer of water a mere two molecules thick can prevent this from occurring. Water is displaced so the molecules involved can spread over the system. Finally, bone strength develops gradually, probably through dipole-dipole interaction.

Bioadhesion involves the linking of side chains of proteins. A study involving dogs showed that certain sugars engender thrombo-

genicity. It has been found that clusters of sugars can form a tree-like structure that presents multiple bonds to the substrate. Though the initial bonds may be non-specific, these are gradually replaced by more specific, stronger bonds. One aim of research is to discover if better molecular detail could provide a way to speed up bone formation and integration.

Subjects for Further Study

Research has to be able to look at initial events of osseointegration that cover a time scale of seconds to weeks, then stretching to years, but for a complete understanding, *in vivo* studies need to look at what cells are present and what is happening. The problem is that the information required is on a scale of less than 1 micrometer. In bone formation, for example, it is known that early formation of calcium carbonate is transformed to hydroxyapatite. Researchers also need to study the mineralization of new generated bone. Generally, *in vivo*, the mineralization response starts with amorphous calcium phosphate, which subsequently mineralizes, with remodeling continuing for more than a year. Researchers know that mechanical factors can come into play and affect whether or not this process may trigger fibrous tissue formation and hinder osseointegration. The process is a complex one and may involve a variety of cells including fibroblasts, osteocytes, osteoblasts, and osteoclasts.

Over the years, researchers have found that osseointegration is a far more tolerant technique than had been originally considered. It has occurred even in compromised tissues. However, lessons have also been learned about factors that can hinder the osseointegration process. For example, if kappa-casein is applied to an implant prior to installation, osseointegration will not happen. Severe infection also prevents bone from developing close apposition to a titanium fixture, though minor infections can be treated so that adequate osseointegration is achieved.

Mechanical overloading at an early stage can also have a detrimental affect on the osseointegration process. Dental bridges using cantilevers have been shown to cause problems, as has biting load distribution governed by the number of fixtures installed. Such effects are controlled by the various cell populations that come into play at different times during the healing and remodeling of bone.

There is no doubt that the growing interest in the cellular and molecular aspects of osseointegration will begin to bear fruit over the next few years. A number of researchers worldwide are seeking to address the gaps in knowledge at this level, and a series of projects have already been initiated that will help unlock the secrets of osseointegration.

12 Training, Communications, and Collaboration

"Delightful task! To rear the tender thought, to teach the young idea how to shoot."

James Thomson, 1700-1748

The preceding three chapters illustrate the tremendous activity that continues in developments and research in osseointegration. This activity is on a global scale and is multidisciplinary in nature. This is no serendipity. From the outset, Per-Ingvar Brånemark believed the support and collaboration of like-minded people around the world would be the way toward the proper development of this technique in all its manifestations.

Original Expansion

When the osseointegration technique was officially approved in Sweden for dentistry, decision makers in the health care system envisioned that the clinical work for dental applications would be carried out at a limited number of dedicated centers around the country. Brånemark personally undertook the training of those select groups of clinicians interested in learning his method. He felt that his personal involvement during those early stages was vital to ensure the strict procedures required for the success of osseointegration for the patient. It was particularly important that clinicians truly understood the need to follow the philosophy of osseointegration and were wholeheartedly committed to it.

Further, the components and equipment necessary to carry out osseointegration procedures were only made available to those who had been appropriately trained by Brånemark and his team. This was an attempt to ensure that only the highest standard of patient treatment and care was maintained. For many years following the commercialization of the system, the company was careful to sell only to those practitioners who had attended approved courses on the Brånemark system.

The almost evangelical approach adopted by Brånemark during the selection and training of other clinicians had a very practical motive. As the dental community in Sweden had been generally hostile to Brånemark's ideas, he felt the future of osseointegration needed to be in the hands of dental surgeons not biased by negative views. In addition, the strict patient follow-up procedures existing within the Swedish health care system would also help verify the clinical success of the technique over the long term. Brånemark says we learn by experience, and experience takes time. There are no shortcuts.

In the light of the perspective that only the passage of years can provide, this approach has been proved appropriate. Brånemark's concern has helped to maintain and support the reputation of osseointegration. It can be compared favorably with the proliferation of competing dental implant systems that do not have the same clinical pedigree and body of scientific evidence behind them.

International Collaboration

Brånemark knew the ability of the technique to stand the scrutiny of peers was also important to learning about ways osseointegration could be further refined, complemented, and developed. He welcomed intellectual input from others interested in working with osseointegration. The founding of the Institute for Applied Biotechnology in 1978 provided the cornerstone of this idea. The Institute was set up as a forum for communication and training, as well as being a link between basic research and clinical applications. It was set up as an independent, non-profit foundation to foster contacts between universities and other research centers. Under this general umbrella, the Brånemark Osseointegration Center was established in Gothenburg in 1989 as a way of expanding and improving osseointegration still further.

Many of Brånemark's initial contacts with international co-workers came from requests to learn about osseointegration following the Toronto conference. So, during the 1980s, Brånemark conducted a number of international training courses. He quickly established close working relationships with a number of groups in the United States, Europe, Australia, and Japan (Fig 12-1). Gradually these relationships deepened into such respect, trust, and collaboration that these pioneering groups who have worked to protect, maintain, and further the developments in osseointegration continue to support and underpin new research. Pioneer centers are located in Boston, Borås, Dublin, Leuven, Malmö, Perth, Seattle, Spokane, and Toronto. These centers are headed by some of the world's most renowned experts in the field of oral and maxillofacial reconstruction. Their considerable stature in these fields has always enhanced the power, integrity, and quality of the research work related to osseointegration.

During the early years, the support of a select group of individuals in carrying out duplicate studies was a vital step in the acceptance of the technique in the wider medical community as a whole. Their continued support and commitment to further research and collaboration continues to guarantee that progress in osseointegration is made. Brånemark has always valued this collaboration highly and, over the years, has developed deep friendships with many of his international colleagues.

It was in 1989 that one of the first centers outside Sweden was established. The European Osseointegration Training Center was established at the Catholic University in Leuven, Belgium, under the leadership of Professor Daniel van Steenberghe. At the time, Steenberghe commented, "Training and experience are essential for proficient work with the Brånemark system." Steenberghe, himself, is a reflection of the tremendous intellects that Brånemark has managed to gather around him to support his work

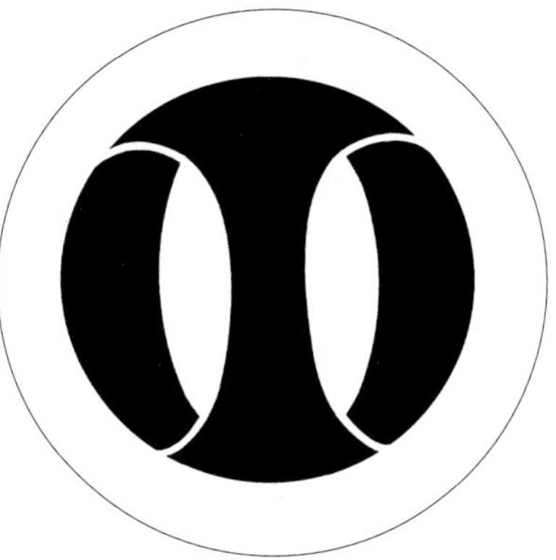

Fig 12-1 This logo was developed to represent osseointegration and is now used as an international symbol by the collaborating centers throughout the world.

on osseointegration. Steenberghe is a significant researcher and clinician in his own field, as well as the work he is involved with on osseointegration. There are many others with equally impressive credentials such as Professor Patrick Henry in Australia and Dr. Kenji Higuchi in the United States who add significantly to the body of expertise required to push forward the knowledge about osseointegration.

In addition, during the 1990s, new Associated Brånemark Osseointegration Centers have joined this growing network. Currently such centers are located in Barcelona and Madrid, Spain; Bauru and São Paulo, Brazil; Santiago, Chile; Marseilles, France; Tokyo, Japan; and Treviso, Italy.

The importance of this network cannot be overestimated. The Associated Brånemark Osseointegration Center based in Barcelona has links with the oral surgery department at the University of Barcelona where center staff teach a 3-year post-graduate course in oral surgery and implantology. The center in Bauru, Brazil is located at the University of Sagrado Coraçáo. This university was one of the first, in 1996, to introduce osseointegration studies at the undergraduate level and has added a Master of Science program to the curriculum. Implant treatment has filled a great need in Brazil, where defects can result in social exclusion (Figs 12-2 to 12-4).

Each center tends to have its own particular interest, as well as providing an international resource. For example, the Associated Brånemark Osseointegration Center based in Treviso, Italy, is involved with a number of research projects such as sinus grafting, growth factors, and eval-

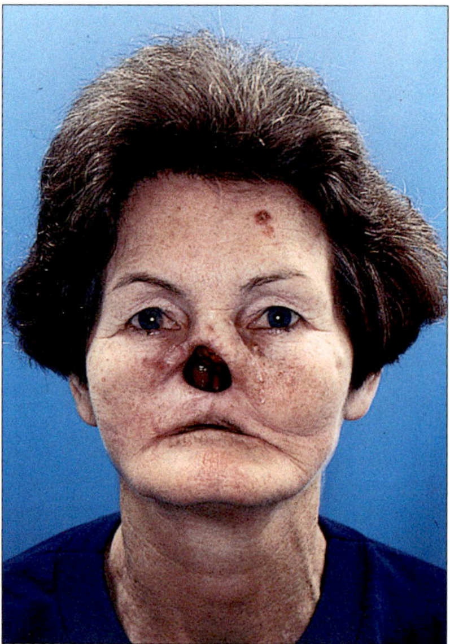

Fig 12-2 This patient was treated in Brazil following loss of teeth, maxillae, and nose resulting from a tumor.

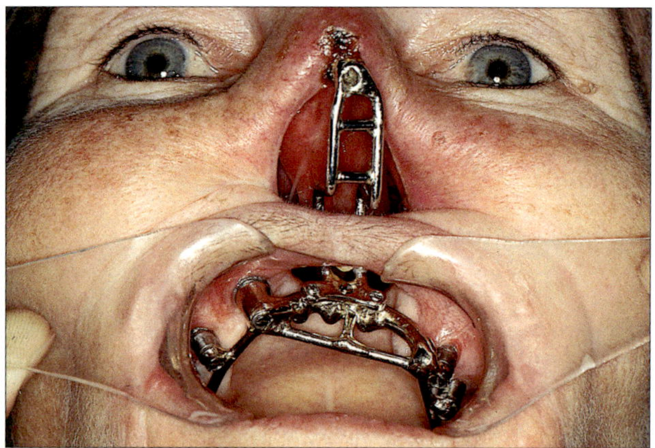

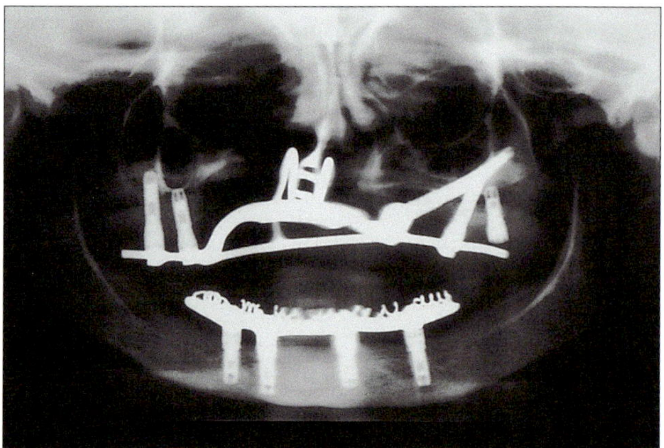

Figs 12-3a and **12-3b** Osseointegration treatment took place in 1992. Internal framework to support dental prosthesis and anchorage point for an artificial nose.

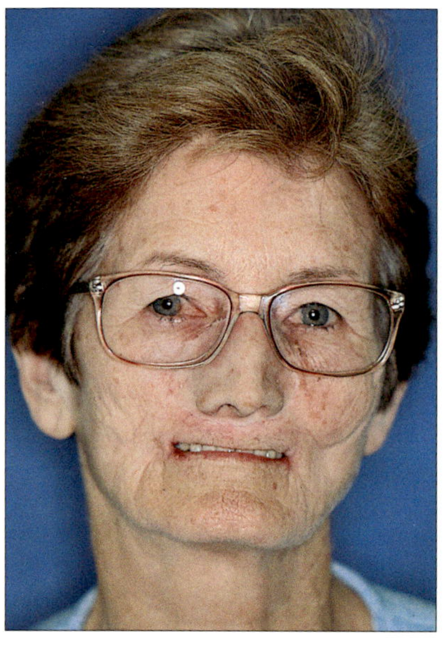

Fig 12-4 The final prosthesis was completed with a pair of glasses. While allowing the patient to eat and talk normally, the prosthesis also enabled her to participate in a full social life.

uation and rehabilitation of extreme bone absorption. The Brazilian center in Bauru has embarked on a program to educate the general public on the potential of the technique and is particularly aiming at the less affluent social classes in the country. Dr. Yataro Komiyama, who heads the equivalent center in Tokyo, has been a prime mover in the introduction of osseointegration throughout Asia, focusing on dental training and patient treatment.

As well as undertaking their own research and treatment activities, all the centers in the network collaborate on international basic and clinical research. They are an important resource when new ideas are moving into clinical reality as they help to provide independently verifiable clinical results based on the treatment of statistically representative numbers of patients. This is a key step toward the commercialization of any development.

The Future of Osseointegration

At a time when there are a growing number of dental implant systems on the market and when the applications of osseointegration are growing, training, research, and communications become increasingly important. There are still many questions to be answered about the basic mechanisms that control osseointegration. Additionally there is more to be done in the refinement and simplification of the technique to reduce further the cost of treatment so it is within the financial reach of all those who could benefit. Then there are the clinical problems to be resolved for applications in orthopedics so that this can be introduced on a wider scale. International collaboration plays a vital role in all these areas.

Collaboration and cooperation with industrial partners and patients are equally as important. In Brånemark's experience, placing patients at the center of care and considering them part of the team reaps enormous benefits for all concerned. The patients feel involved in their treatment, feel part of the decision-making process related to their rehabilitation, and are confident about outcomes because they are well informed about the procedures. For the clinicians, there is

increased satisfaction related to having happy patients, and for those carrying out more challenging procedures, the information and feedback gained from patients can be of enormous value for developing and refining procedures.

Finally the nature of osseointegration means that certain prerequisites are demanded to ensure the long-term survival of such fixtures in living bone and tissue. It depends on constant vigilance to ensure the quality of such components and instruments. Also, it means modifications and changes to either production methods or component design have to be based on clinical experience and proven methodologies.

This puts a tremendous responsibility on any medical equipment company involved in the manufacture of such components. A medical equipment company cannot afford to ignore clinical experience and research results of those involved in the provision of medical services and the further development and refinement of osseointegration. Cooperating with researchers has many benefits for industrial companies. It supports their own understanding so they can understand their customers better, with the hope of delivering suitably tailored services and products. Such collaboration also enhances a company's reputation, as well as benefiting sales and long-term growth if associated with well-known experts in their fields. Researchers and industry have clear roles to play but with an overriding responsibility to the patient.

Osseointegration is a technique with a long-term future. Many potential clinical applications of osseointegration still have some issues to be resolved, but this is only a matter of time (Fig 12-5). In the last few years, China has become interested in learning about the technology, and Brånemark has made a number of visits there to give lectures and demonstrations. With this country's interest, commitment, resources, and need, it may be possible to establish osseointegration at a level not achieved today. Already osseointegration has had a profound impact on individuals throughout the world, yet much is still to be done. It remains an exciting and often frustrating field in which to work, but the rewards in terms of its ability to transform the lives of patients are significant. What will be achieved in the future will continue to depend on the energies of individuals working together

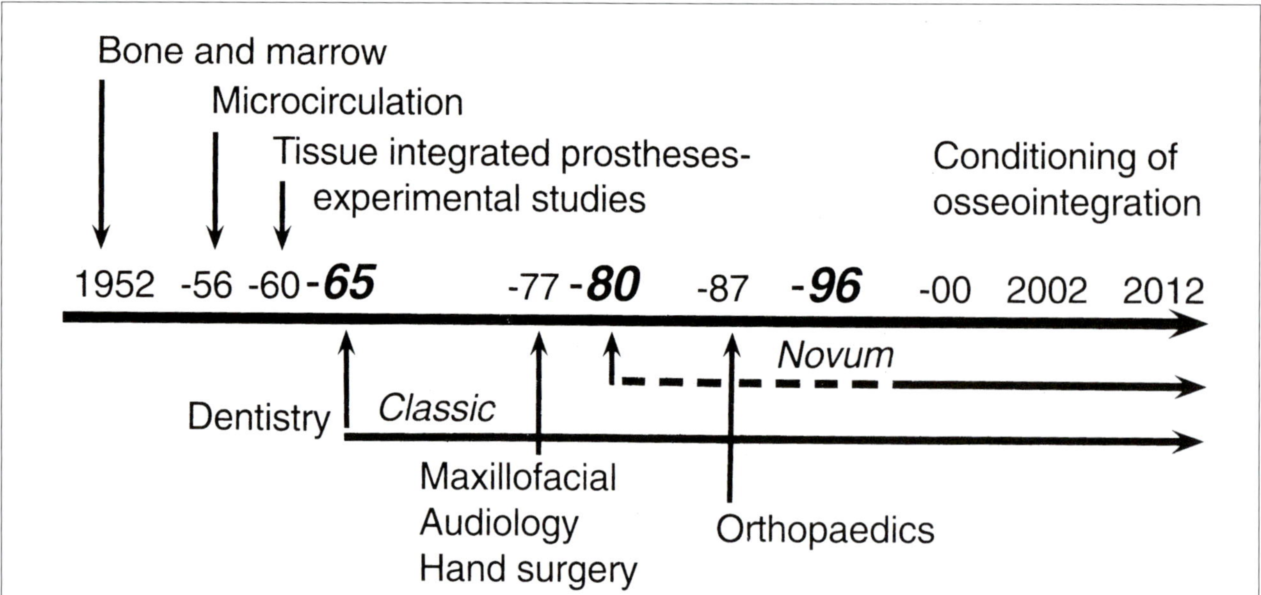

Fig 12-5 Timeline of developments in osseointegration. How quickly new clinical applications develop will be based on the combined efforts of the health care systems, clinicians, and industry.

for the good of each patient who might benefit. In 2001, Brånemark retired from the active administration of the Institute, but it is highly unlikely that his energy and imagination for applying osseointegration to the benefit of patients will diminish.

Bibliography

Albrektsson T. Osseointegration of bone implants: A review of an alternative mode of fixation. Acta Orthop Scand 1987;58:567–577.

Albrektsson T, Zarb G. The Brånemark Osseointegrated Implant. Chicago: Quintessence, 1989.

Alexander W, Street A. Metals in the Service of Man, ed 9. Harmondsworth: Pelican, 1989.

Bone-Anchored Implants in the Head and Neck Region. Swedish Council on Technology Assessment in Health Care. Report from a conference, Gothenburg, 1 Sept 1988.

Brånemark P-I. Intravascular Anatomy of Blood Cells in Man. Basel, Switzerland: S. Karger, 1971.

Brånemark P-I, Albrektsson T, Zarb G (eds). Tissue-Integrated Prostheses: Osseointegration in Clinical Dentistry. Chicago: Quintessence, 1985.

Brånemark P-I, Oliveira MF (eds). Craniofacial Prostheses: Anaplastology and Osseointegration. Chicago: Quintessence, 1997.

Brånemark P-I, Rydevik BL, Skalak R (eds). Osseointegration in Skeletal Reconstruction and Joint Replacement: Second International Workshop on Osseointegration in Skeletal Reconstruction and Joint Replacement, Rancho Santa Fe, California, 27–29 October 1994.

Brånemark R. A Biomechanical Study of Osseointegration [thesis]. Gothenburg: Gothenburg University, 1996.

Carlsson P. On Direct Bone Conduction Hearing Devices, Technical Report 195. Chalmers: Department of Applied Electronics, Chalmers University of Technology, 1990.

Cowan K. Implant and Transplant Surgery. London: Murray, 1971.

Holgers KM. Soft Tissue Reactions Around Clinical Skin-Penetrating Implants [thesis]. Gothenburg: Gothenburg University, 1994.

Johns RB. A Study of the Response of Tissue to Endodontic and Endosseous Implants in *Macaca irus* Monkeys [thesis]. London: London University, 1973.

Kasemo B, Lausmaa J. Biomaterial and implant surfaces: On the role of cleanliness, contamination and preparation procedures. J Biomed Mater Res 1988;22(A2 suppl):145–158.

Kasemo B, Lausmaa J. The biomaterial-tissue interface and its analogues in surface science and technology. Presented at the Non-Biomaterial Interface Conference, Toronto, December 1990.

Lekholm U, Ericsson I, Adell R, Slots J. The condition of the soft tissues at tooth and fixture abutments supporting fixed bridges: A microbiological and histological study. J Clin Periodontol 1986;13:558–562.

Lundborg G. Hand Surgery: An Introduction [student literature]. Lund, Sweden: Lund University, 1988.

Lundborg G. Nerve Injury and Repair. New York: Churchill Livingstone, 1988.

Mylanus EAM. The Bone Anchored Hearing Aid: Clinical and Audiological Aspects [thesis]. Nijmegen: Catholic University of Nijmegen, 1994.

Rhodes P. An Outline History of Medicine. London: Butterworths, 1985.

Skalak R, Zhao Y. Interaction of force-fitting and surface roughness of implants. Clin Implant Dent Relat Res 2000;2:219–224.

Skalak R, Zhao Y. Similarity of stress distribution in bone for various implant surface roughness heights of similar form. Clin Implant Dent Relat Res 2000;2:225–230.

Williams E. A Matter of Balance. Gothenburg: Akademiförlaget, 1992.

Williams E, Rydevik B, Johns R, Brånemark P-I (eds). Osseoperception and Musculo-Skeletal Function. Gothenburg: Institute of Applied Biotechnology, 1999.

Williams E (ed). From Molecules to Man. Gothenburg: Institute of Applied Biotechnology, 1999.

Zarb G, Schmitt A, Baker G. Tissue-integrated prosthesis: Osseointegrated research in Toronto. Int J Periodontics Restorative Dent 1987;7(1):8–35.

Illustration Credits

Fig 1-1 Brånemark P-I (ed). The Brånemark Novum Protocol for Same-Day Teeth: A Global Perspective. Berlin: Quintessenz, 2001.

Fig 1-2 Brånemark R. A Biomechanical Study of Osseointegration: In Vivo Measurements in Rat, Rabbit, Dog and Man [doctoral dissertation]. Gothenburg: Gothenburg University, 1996.

Fig 1-3 Courtesy of P-I Brånemark.

Figs 1-4 to 1-6 Brånemark P-I. Intravascular Anatomy of Blood Cells in Man. Basel, Switzerland: Karger, 1971.

Fig 1-7 Brånemark P-I. Capillary form and function. The microcirculation of granulation tissue. Bibl Anat 1965;7:9-28.

Fig 2-1 Courtesy of P-I Brånemark.

Fig 2-2 Brånemark P-I, Hansson BO, Adell R, Breine U, Lindstrom J, Hallen O, Ohman A. Osseointegrated implants in the treatment of the edentulous jaw. Experience from a 10-year period. Scand J Plast Reconstr Surg Suppl 1977;16:1–132. Used with permission.

Fig 2-3 Courtesy of P-I Brånemark.

Fig 2-4 Courtesy of P-I Brånemark.

Fig 2-5 Courtesy of P-I Brånemark.

Fig 2-6 Courtesy of the Institute for Applied Biotechnology.

Fig 3-1 Courtesy of the Institute for Applied Biotechnology.

Fig 3-2 Courtesy of the Institute for Applied Biotechnology.

Fig 3-3 Williams E, Rydevik B, Brånemark P-I (eds). Osseointegration from Molecule to Man. Gothenburg: Institute for Applied Biotechnology, 2000:87. Courtesy of the Institute for Applied Biotechnology.

Figs 4-1 to 4-6 Williams E, Rydevik B, Brånemark P-I (eds). Osseointegration from Molecule to Man. Gothenburg: Institute for Applied Biotechnology, 2000. Courtesy of the Institute for Applied Biotechnology.

Fig 5-1 Courtesy of P-I Brånemark.

Figs 5-2a to 5-2c Tjellström A, Jansson K, Brånemark P-I. Craniofacial defects. In: Worthington P, Brånemark P-I (eds). Advanced Osseointegration Surgery: Applications in the Maxillofacial Region. Chicago: Quintessence, 1992: 293–312. Used with permission.

Figs 5-2d and 5-2e Courtesy of P-I Brånemark.

Figs 5-3a to 5-3j Courtesy of P-I Brånemark.

Figs 6-1 to 6-4 Courtesy of P-I Brånemark.

Fig 7-1 Courtesy of the Institute for Applied Biotechnology.

Fig 7-2 Williams E. A Matter of Balance. Gothenburg: Akademiförlaget, 1992.

Figs 7-3a and 7-3b Courtesy of P-I Brånemark.

Figs 7-4a to 7-4c Williams E, Rydevik B, Johns R, Brånemark P-I (eds). Osseoperception and Musculo-Skeletal Function. Gothenburg: Institute of Applied Biotechnology, 1999. Courtesy of the Institute of Applied Biotechnology.

Figs 7-5 to 7-8 Courtesy of P-I Brånemark.

Fig 8-3 Courtesy of the Institute for Applied Biotechnology.

Fig 8-4 Courtesy of P-I Brånemark.

Fig 9-1 Courtesy of the Institute for Applied Biotechnology.

Fig 9-2 Haraldson T, Carlsson GE, Ingervall B. Functional state, bite force and postural muscle activity in patients with osseointegrated oral implant bridges. Acta Odontol Scand 1979;37:195–206.

Fig 9-3 Lundqvist S, Haraldson T. Occusal perception of thickness in patients with bridges on osseointegrated oral implants. Scand J Dent Res 1984;92:88–92.

Figs 9-4a and 9-4b Courtesy of P-I Brånemark.

Figs 9-5 and 9-6 Williams E, Rydevik B, Johns R, Brånemark P-I (eds). Osseoperception and Musculo-Skeletal Function. Gothenburg: Institute of Applied Biotechnology, 1999. Courtesy of the Institute of Applied Biotechnology.

Fig 10-1 Courtesy of the Institute of Applied Biotechnology.

Fig 10-2 Haraldson T. A photoelastic study of some biomechanical factors affecting the anchorage of osseointegrated implants in the jaw. Scand J Plast Reconstr Surg 1980;14: 209–214.

Figs 10-3 and 10-4 Courtesy of P-I Brånemark.

Fig 10-5 Brånemark R. A Biomechanical Study of Osseointegration: In Vivo Measurements in Rat, Rabbit, Dog and Man [doctoral dissertation]. Gothenburg: Gothenburg University, 1996.

Figs 10-6 and **10-7** Courtesy of P-I Brånemark.

Fig 10-8 Brånemark P-I (ed). The Brånemark Novum Protocol for Same-Day Teeth: A Global Perspective. Berlin: Quintessenz, 2001.

Fig 11-1 Courtesy of the Institute of Applied Biotechnology.

Figs 12-1 to 12-5 Courtesy of the Institute of Applied Biotechnology.